The "I LOVE MY INSTANT POT®" Keto Diet

Recipe Book

From *Poached Eggs* to *Quick Chicken Parmesan*,
175 Fat-Burning Keto Recipes

Sam Dillard of HeyKetoMama.com

Use of the trademarks is authorized by DOUBLE INSIGHT Inc., owner of Instant Pot®.

Adams Media
New York   London   Toronto   Sydney   New Delhi

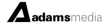

Adams Media
An Imprint of Simon & Schuster, Inc.
57 Littlefield Street
Avon, Massachusetts 02322

First Adams Media trade paperback edition July 2018

ADAMS MEDIA and colophon are trademarks of Simon & Schuster.

For information about special discounts for bulk purchases, please contact Simon & Schuster Special Sales at 1-866-506-1949 or business@simonandschuster.com.

The Simon & Schuster Speakers Bureau can bring authors to your live event. For more information or to book an event contact the Simon & Schuster Speakers Bureau at 1-866-248-3049 or visit our website at www.simonspeakers.com.

Interior design by Colleen Cunningham
Photographs by James Stefiuk

Manufactured in the United States of America

10 9 8 7 6 5 4 3 2 1

Library of Congress Cataloging-in-Publication Data
Dillard, Sam, author.
The "I love my instant pot®" keto diet recipe book / Sam Dillard of HeyKetoMama.com.
Avon, Massachusetts: Adams Media, 2018.
Series: "I love my" series.
Includes index.
LCCN 2018003626 (print) | LCCN 2018011036 (ebook) | ISBN 9781507207680 (pb) | ISBN 9781507207697 (ebook)
LCSH: Reducing diets--Recipes. | Ketogenic diet. | Quick and easy cooking. | BISAC: COOKING / Health & Healing / Low Carbohydrate. | COOKING / Methods / Special Appliances. | HEALTH & FITNESS / Diets. | LCGFT: Cookbooks.
LCC RM222.2 (ebook) | LCC RM222.2 .D575 2018 (print) | DDC 641.5/63--dc23
LC record available at https://lccn.loc.gov/2018003626

ISBN 978-1-5072-0768-0
ISBN 978-1-5072-0769-7 (ebook)

The information in this book should not be used for diagnosing or treating any health problem. Not all diet and exercise plans suit everyone. You should always consult a trained medical professional before starting a diet, taking any form of medication, or embarking on any fitness or weight-training program. The author and publisher disclaim any liability arising directly or indirectly from the use of this book.

Always follow safety and commonsense cooking protocols while using kitchen utensils, operating ovens and stoves, and handling uncooked food. If children are assisting in the preparation of any recipe, they should always be supervised by an adult.

Thank you to my family and friends for your kind words.

Joey and Maya, your infinite hugs.
Joe, your endless encouragement.

This book is for my mom, who never thought I was listening
to her cooking lessons for all those years.

To my fellow ketoers, KCKO.

Contents

Introduction

You may be wondering what the hype is about the Instant Pot®. Or, maybe you already have an Instant Pot® and use it nearly every day. If you're like me, once you discover how versatile and easy Instant Pot® cooking is, you'll be hooked. So, why does everyone love the Instant Pot®?

It's the perfect appliance if you love cooking, but simply don't have a lot of time. It has multiple features all in one pot that make prepping with (and washing!) multiple pans outdated. The Instant Pot® can sauté, slow cook, and of course, prepare meals in a fraction of the time. It's the solution for every busy person who needs to make healthy home-cooked meals. You may be reading this as a fellow low-carber, or as someone who is interested in learning more and wondering if a ketogenic diet is right for you. The ketogenic diet is a very low-carbohydrate, high-fat, adequate-protein diet. I like to think of it less as a fad diet and more of a lifestyle that focuses on overall health and eating real food. On a ketogenic diet, you get most of your calories from fat. This may seem confusing, as it is different from the standard American diet where a balance of carbs and protein make up the bulk of our nutrition, with fats being allowed in small portions. There are many benefits to a ketogenic diet such as appetite suppression and weight loss, but keto has also been promising in treating diabetes, epilepsy, and other autoimmune disorders that are affected by fluctuating insulin levels.

The Instant Pot® and the ketogenic diet go hand in hand. When you cut out excessively processed foods that are loaded with carbs, it can be a bit overwhelming to find yourself cooking wholesome meals every day. Real foods are better for your body, but they generally take longer to prepare—and that's tough with a busy schedule. The Instant Pot® makes that task much faster and much more fun! Also, many people who follow a ketogenic diet like to meal prep for a whole week at a time by cooking in large batches. Sometimes the thing that keeps you on track is knowing you have a nutritious meal ready in the fridge, or that you can whip one up in just about 20 minutes. Let the Instant Pot® help you with that!

Throughout this book you'll learn everything you need to know about how and why to use the Instant Pot® as well as some basics that will help you find success following the ketogenic diet. Let's get cooking!

Cooking with an Instant Pot®

Learning to use a pressure cooker can feel intimidating at first, but trust me, you'll get the hang of it in no time. In fact, you'll soon wonder how you ever lived without it. This chapter will introduce you to all the Instant Pot® buttons, explain how and when to release pressure from the Instant Pot®, teach you how to keep the Instant Pot® clean, and tell you about some accessories that can take your pressure cooking to the next level.

While this chapter will cover the basics of using your Instant Pot®, the first step is reading the manual that came with your Instant Pot®. Learning how to use the Instant Pot® thoroughly is the key to success and will familiarize you with trouble-shooting issues as well as safety functions. Reading over the manual and doing the water test run will help you feel more confident. Confidence in the kitchen is what ultimately leads to success in creating delicious meals.

Why Pressure Cooking?

Pressure cooking has always been popular, but with today's electric pressure cookers like the Instant Pot®, it's easier than ever to do. Here are some reasons the Instant Pot® will become your favorite appliance:

It's fast and convenient: You can spend less time in the kitchen cooking, without sacrificing flavor. This is especially helpful if you like to prepare your meals ahead of time in large batches.

It's smart: Ever put dinner in the oven, then run off to do something else around the house and forget to go back when it's done? The Instant Pot® has you covered! It will automatically switch into Keep Warm mode once the timer goes off. No more burnt meals!

It uses less energy: We all use the oven to cook too, but it definitely comes with a price. Besides heating up the house during the warm months, it can take hours to slow roast large cuts of meat, and that takes its toll on your home's energy consumption. The Instant Pot® can perform the same functions as a stove and a slow cooker in less time, meaning less energy output.

There's less cleanup: Who wants to clean half a dozen pans after a meal? The Instant Pot® one-pot technique means minimal cleanup...and more time to do other things!

Now let's take a closer look at all of the ways the Instant Pot® can prepare food.

The Functions of an Instant Pot®

As soon as you see the buttons on the Instant Pot®, you'll see the amazing range of tasks this tool can handle—it can steam veggies, cook a whole chicken, and even make a smooth, delicious New York–style cheesecake.

The key is knowing how the cooking programs work on the Instant Pot® and when to use them. Once you have a basic understanding of the functions, you'll be well on your way to creating your favorite Instant Pot® meal in just the push of a button.

Following are the buttons you will most frequently use when cooking foods on the ketogenic diet. (Not all the Instant Pot® buttons will be utilized in this particular book. There are different Instant Pot® models available, but all versions have the basic functions mentioned in these recipes.)

Manual: This will likely be your most used button. It allows you to manually program the pressure level and cooking time. The +/- keys adjust the cooking time, and the Pressure button toggles between High Pressure and Low Pressure (High Pressure is the default). This button makes it easy to get your Instant Pot® started without much thought, especially once you're more comfortable with determining cook times.

Steam: This button allows you to steam meats and vegetables. Steaming is an excellent way to cook because it allows the food to retain nutrients and keep a fresh flavor. The Adjust button allows you to choose 3 to 15 minutes of cooking. The quick-release option will prevent your fresh veggies from getting soggy.

Slow Cook: This button allows the Instant Pot® to function as a slow cooker. This non-pressure cooking method allows your Instant Pot® to cook while being temperature controlled, similar to a slow cooker. The Low, Normal, and More options correspond to a slow cooker's Low, Medium, and High settings. (Your slow cooker's glass lid might fit if you want to be able to see in while you cook this way.)

Soup/Broth: This Instant Pot® mode can be adjusted depending on your soup contents. You can even sauté your onions and garlic right in the pot before adding the rest of your ingredients and going into a pressure cooking program.

Meat/Stew: This button allows you to cook savory roasts, fall-off-the-bone ribs, hearty stews, and more in less time than using the oven. The mode can be adjusted based on meat texture and the timer can be adjusted to increase time based on the type and size of the meat.

Egg: This button allows you to cook boiled eggs quickly and easily. The mode can be adjusted to reflect your preference with soft-, medium-, or hard-boiled eggs. Since you actually steam the eggs rather than boil them, they are less likely to overcook and more likely to have fluffy yolks. Not to mention, they take less than 10 minutes and you don't have to watch them.

Sauté: This button helps you save time and add flavor to your meal before you begin a pressure cooking program. It allows you to pan-sear, stir-fry, and simmer to reduce liquids. With this function, it is important that you do *not* use the lid.

Cake: This button allows you to cook moist cakes and even perfect cheesecakes. The modes allow you to choose a light or dense cake. The More function allows you to make creamy New York–style cheesecake—it will never crack or dry out!

Keep Warm/Cancel: When the Instant Pot® is programmed, this button ends the cooking program and places it into standby mode. The Keep Warm function is automatically enabled after a cooking program but it can be turned off by pressing the program key you used to turn it on again. You will know it worked because the Stay Warm indicator light will turn off.

Locking and Pressure-Release Methods

Locking the lid of the Instant Pot® is very easy but it's important to do properly. The lid fits in place on the pot, and when rotated 30 degrees clockwise, makes a small sound to let you know the position has been changed.

As the Instant Pot® builds pressure, a red indicator will pop up to let you know that it is fully pressurized and ready to start counting down the timer. Sometimes this is accompanied by a little hiss of steam, but it should be relatively quiet. The amount of time it takes

for the pressure to be reached depends on the length of the cooking program.

There are three ways to release pressure from the Instant Pot®, and then you can remove the lid.

Natural Release

The Instant Pot® will naturally release pressure after a cooking program has completed. The time this will take varies based on how long the meal has been cooking. Once the pressure indicator drops, you may take off the lid. Never force the lid off if it will not turn, or attempt to take it off during a cooking program. (Refer to the manual if needed.) Allowing a natural pressure release is great for recipes with meat because it allows the meat to remain tender and retain moisture. Some recipes may call for a timed natural release followed by a quick release, while others require a fully natural release.

Quick Release

To do a quick release, once the cooking program has completed, carefully turn the valve from Sealing to Venting to allow the steam to release. Be sure to stand back from the Instant Pot® as you do this and keep your hands clear of the steam. A quick release is ideal for steamed vegetables because it helps prevent overcooking. A quick release usually takes 1–2 minutes.

Pulse Release

The pulse release is a combination of natural and quick releases. You wait a certain amount of time before venting the remaining pressure.

Opening the Lid

Once the pressure indicator has dropped (regardless of which method you use), you may remove the lid. Simply turn the lid counterclockwise until it makes a sound indicating it is fully in the open position and aligns with the Open arrow. If the lid will not turn, double-check that the pressure is fully released, and the red valve indicator has dropped down.

Pot-in-Pot Accessories

Pot-in-pot accessories are those that fit inside the Instant Pot®, usually placed on the steam rack, while water is added to the bottom. (Every Instant Pot® comes with a steam rack, a metal piece that is placed in the bottom of the pot and elevates food.) These accessories can broaden the number of recipes you can make in the Instant Pot® and open up a new world of exciting possibilities.

Steamer basket: You can set veggies on the steam rack to cook, but nothing can beat the convenience of a great steamer basket. A steamer basket will make removing veggies a breeze and also comes in handy when you want to cook a dozen eggs or steam chicken or fish.

Ramekins: Small 4-inch ramekins are perfect for making mini cakes and quiches. If they're oven-safe, they're safe to use in the Instant Pot®.

Springform pan: A 7-inch springform pan fits perfectly into the 8-quart Instant Pot®. If you have a smaller Instant Pot®, use a 4-inch springform pan.

Cake pan: A 6- or 7-inch round cake pan makes the perfect-sized cake for 4–6 people without excessive leftovers.

Glass bowl: A 7-cup glass bowl fits perfectly in the Instant Pot® and is ideal for cooking delicate ingredients such as eggs and seafood.

Silicone baking cups: These versatile cups are great for making mini meatloaves, muffins, and other baked goods. They're inexpensive and can even go straight to the freezer after cooking.

Glass Mason jars: As though Mason jars don't have enough uses around the kitchen, they also work great in the Instant Pot®. If you don't have ramekins you can use them for quiches or even personal-sized mug cakes, or yogurt, if your Instant Pot® has that feature. Just be sure to never use the lid on the Mason jar in the Instant Pot®.

Accessory Removal

These tools will help you take items out of the Instant Pot® safely and easily.

Tongs: These will be helpful when lifting meat in and out of the Instant Pot®. Tongs are also helpful when removing steamer baskets.

Small kitchen towel: Sometimes a simple kitchen towel can be the best tool. From wiping condensation away to taking out a foil-covered pan, these are always great to have around.

Aluminum foil sling: You can make a sling out of foil to set under pans to help them lift out of the Instant Pot® more easily. This is a good method for removing cooking dishes that may spill or items such as cheesecakes that require gentle removal.

Cleaning the Instant Pot®

Before cleaning, ensure that your Instant Pot® is completely cool and unplugged.

Inner pot, steam rack, lid, and included accessories: All these parts are dishwasher safe, but use the top rack for the lid. You can also hand-wash in hot, soapy water.

Heating unit: It's unlikely that this area will accumulate much grime, but wiping the inner pot with a damp cloth will keep it clean. Do not submerge in water.

Lid: The lid can be disassembled to be cleaned. The sealing ring can be removed and washed with soap and water. The pressure-release handle can be popped out and washed to ensure there are no particles causing blockage. The anti-block shield (the small basket under the lid) should be removed and cleaned regularly with soap and water. It blocks food from entering the pressure-release valve.

The outside: Wipe the outside and the inside lid of the Instant Pot® with a damp cloth.

After it's all clean, be sure all components are put back in the correct position before beginning your next cooking adventure.

What Is a Ketogenic Diet?

The ketogenic diet, or keto, is a very low-carb, moderate-protein, and high-fat diet that allows the body to fuel itself without the use of glucose or high levels of carbohydrates. When the body is in short supply of glucose, ketones are made in the liver from the breakdown of fats through a process called ketosis. (Please note that this differs from ketoacidosis.) With careful tracking, creative meals, and self-control, this diet can lead to weight loss, lower blood sugar, regulated insulin levels, and controlled cravings.

When you eat a very high-carb diet (pizza, pasta, breads, pastries), your body takes those carbs and turns them into glucose to power itself. When you cut out the carbs, your metabolism burns fat instead. Typically, a ketogenic diet restricts carbs to between 0–50 grams per day.

What Are Macros?

Macronutrients, or macros, are the three ways our bodies produce energy. They include carbohydrates, protein, and fat. When you're following keto, it is very important to track how many grams of each macronutrient you consume each day:

Carbs: around 5 percent of your daily calories

Protein: around 25 percent of your daily calories

Healthy fats: around 70 percent of your daily calories

Some of the best-quality fats come from natural sources such as fish, avocados, and nuts. These fats can help reduce your cholesterol, keep your heart strong, and fuel your body throughout the day. You should always beware of unhealthy fats, however, that can come from foods like cookies and french fries. Overconsumption of these, especially in conjunction with a high-carb diet, can contribute to heart disease, low energy, and unwanted weight gain.

Net Carbs versus Total Carbs

Most people following keto opt to track net carbs instead of total carbs. You can figure that out by subtracting your dietary fiber intake from your total carb intake:

Total carbs minus dietary fiber equals net carbs.

You may also subtract sugar alcohols (listed on nutritional labels under the carbohydrate count) from the total carb count. Net is generally the preferred method because of how your body reacts to the fiber and sugar alcohols. On nutrition labels, the grams of dietary fiber and sugar alcohols are already included in the total carb count, but because fiber and (some) sugar alcohols are carbs that your body can't digest, they have no effect on your blood sugar levels and can be subtracted.

Top Ketogenic Tips to Remember

Finally, keep these quick tips in mind as you plan your daily meals.

Carbs are a limit: Don't go above your allotted daily net carbs.

Protein is a goal: This is the most important macro to hit. If you're losing weight, you want to make sure you're eating enough protein to keep you from also losing muscle.

Fat is a lever: In this diet, fat is designed to keep you full. If you're hungry, go ahead and eat that healthy fat up to your limit. If you're not hungry, you don't have to hit your fat macros.

With the quick and easy recipes in this book, you should never feel deprived on your keto journey. Just remember, if you fall off the wagon, the most important thing is to get back on as quickly as possible. Allow yourself grace and time, but never give up just because you slipped up.

Now that you have a better understanding of your Instant Pot® and the ketogenic diet, let's get cooking! You'll find plenty of recipes to suit all tastes. Use these recipes as a guide and always feel free to season intuitively and customize dishes to your liking.

2

Breakfast

Get ready to make over your mornings with easy, healthy pressure cooking! These recipes will have you full, focused, and ready to take on the day. We all know how important it is to start your day with a nutritious breakfast, but let's face it… that's definitely easier said than done. When you're faced with the reality of your busy morning, you might just find yourself rushing out the door without any solid nourishment. We all know how this story goes: an hour later you're sitting at work starving and searching for a snack.

Skipping breakfast can be a gateway to mindless calorie consumption, but thankfully the Instant Pot® is here to save the day! The meals in this chapter are nutritious and very quick to make. Many of them you can even prepare the night before, so everything is ready to go when you wake up. Once you get into the habit of cooking these meals, your days will seem easier and your body will thank you!

Easy-Prep Egg Muffins

Mornings can be crazy, but these egg bites will give you enough protein to keep your body fueled. These are easy to customize by adding veggies, cooked meat, and your favorite dose of healthy fat. For example, top these with avocado, bacon crumbles—or both! They keep well in the fridge so whenever you need a boost, you'll know a quick and healthy bite is already waiting for you.

- **Hands-on time: 5 minutes**
- **Cook time: 10 minutes**

Serves 6

4 eggs
2 tablespoons heavy cream
¼ teaspoon salt
⅛ teaspoon pepper
⅓ cup shredded cheddar
1 cup water

1 In large bowl, whisk eggs and heavy cream. Add salt and pepper.

2 Pour mixture into 6 silicone cupcake baking molds. Sprinkle cheese into each cup.

3 Pour water into Instant Pot® and place steam rack in bottom of pot. Carefully set filled silicone molds steadily on steam rack. If all do not fit, separate into two batches.

4 Click lid closed. Press the Manual button and adjust time for 10 minutes. When timer beeps, allow a quick release and remove lid. Egg bites will look puffy at first, but will become smaller once they begin to cool. Serve warm.

CALORIES: 90
FAT: 6.5 grams
PROTEIN: 5.8 grams
SODIUM: 186 milligrams
FIBER: 0.0 grams
CARBOHYDRATES: 0.5 grams
NET CARBOHYDRATES: 0.5 grams
SUGAR: 0.3 grams

Individual Mini Quiche

This quiche is perfect for those slow mornings when you have time to start your day in a relaxed way. It's fluffy, flavorful, and full of nourishment. You can mix the ingredients right in the ramekin, so you won't bog down your morning with a sink full of dishes. The next time you have overnight guests, this meal could make a great DIY bar, complete with savory mix-ins.

- **Hands-on time:** 5 minutes
- **Cook time:** 15 minutes

Serves 1

2 eggs
1 tablespoon heavy cream
1 tablespoon diced green pepper
1 tablespoon diced red onion
¼ cup chopped fresh spinach
½ teaspoon salt
¼ teaspoon pepper
1 cup water

1 In medium bowl whisk together all ingredients except water. Pour into 4-inch ramekin. Generally, if the ramekin is oven-safe, it is also safe to use in pressure cooking.

2 Pour water into Instant Pot®. Place steam rack into pot. Carefully place ramekin onto steam rack. Click lid closed. Press the Manual button and set time for 15 minutes. When timer beeps, quick-release the pressure. Serve warm.

CALORIES: 201
PROTEIN: 13.3 grams
FIBER: 0.6 grams
NET CARBOHYDRATES: 2.5 grams
FAT: 14.0 grams
SODIUM: 1,314 milligrams
CARBOHYDRATES: 3.1 grams
SUGAR: 1.5 grams

CUSTOMIZE IT!
You can add your favorite toppings to make your quiche even more delicious. Try adding slices of avocado, a sprinkle of cheese, or a dash of hot sauce for a bold flavor punch.

Cauliflower Breakfast Casserole

If you've been missing hash browns since going keto, you'll love this! The versatile cauliflower will help fill you up, and give you that traditional breakfast taste you desire. Even better, unlike the potatoes you would use to make hash browns, this dish is loaded with nutrients—*not* empty calories. This quick and easy dish is perfect for holidays or family get-togethers.

- **Hands-on time:** 5 minutes
- **Cook time:** 10 minutes

Serves 6

1 cup water
½ head cauliflower, chopped into bite-sized pieces
4 slices bacon
1 pound breakfast sausage
4 tablespoons melted butter
10 eggs
⅓ cup heavy cream
2 teaspoons salt
1 teaspoon pepper
2 tablespoons hot sauce
2 stalks green onion
1 cup shredded sharp cheddar

1 Pour water into Instant Pot® and place steamer basket in bottom. Add cauliflower. Click lid closed.

2 Press the Steam button and adjust time for 1 minute. When timer beeps, quick-release the pressure and place cauliflower to the side in medium bowl.

3 Drain water from Instant Pot®, clean, and replace. Press the Sauté button. Press the Adjust button to set heat to Less. Cook bacon until crispy. Once fully cooked, set aside on paper towels. Add breakfast sausage to pot and brown (still using the Sauté function).

4 While sausage is cooking, whisk butter, eggs, heavy cream, salt, pepper, and hot sauce.

5 When sausage is fully cooked, pour egg mixture into Instant Pot®. Gently stir using silicone spatula until eggs are completely cooked and fluffy. Press the Cancel button.

6 Slice green onions. Sprinkle green onions, bacon, and cheese over mixture and let melt. Serve warm.

CALORIES: 620
PROTEIN: 29.8 grams
FIBER: 1.2 grams
NET CARBOHYDRATES: 3.5 grams

FAT: 49.6 grams
SODIUM: 1,746 milligrams
CARBOHYDRATES: 4.7 grams
SUGAR: 1.7 grams

Simple Hard-Boiled Eggs

Fast, fluffy, and versatile, these hard-boiled eggs are the perfect addition to your mornings. You can create a number of dishes, such as deviled eggs or egg salad, or even add sliced eggs to a salad for an extra boost of protein.

- **Hands-on time:** 1 minute
- **Cook time:** 8 minutes

Serves 12

1 cup water
12 eggs

Place steamer basket or steam rack in bottom of Instant Pot®. Add water. Place eggs in steamer basket. Click lid closed. Press the Egg button. Adjust time to 8 minutes. When timer beeps, quick-release and remove steamer basket.

CALORIES: 77
PROTEIN: 6.3 grams
FIBER: 0.0 grams
NET CARBOHYDRATES: 0.6 grams

FAT: 4.4 grams
SODIUM: 62 milligrams
CARBOHYDRATES: 0.6 grams
SUGAR: 0.6 grams

Greens Power Bowl

Lean, green, and full of protein, this bowl is designed to get you pumped up and ready to attack your day. It has a great balance of healthy fats and micronutrients.

- **Hands-on time:** 10 minutes
- **Cook time:** 10 minutes

Serves 1

1 cup water
2 eggs
1 tablespoon coconut oil
1 tablespoon butter
1 ounce sliced almonds
1 cup fresh spinach, sliced into strips
½ cup kale, sliced into strips
½ clove garlic, minced
½ teaspoon salt
⅛ teaspoon pepper
½ avocado, sliced
⅛ teaspoon red pepper flakes

1 Pour water into Instant Pot® and place steam rack on bottom. Place eggs on steam rack. Click lid closed. Press the Egg button and adjust time for 6 minutes. When timer beeps, quick-release the pressure. Set eggs aside.

2 Pour water out, clean pot, and replace. Press the Sauté button and add coconut oil, butter, and almonds. Sauté for 2–3 minutes until butter begins to turn golden and almonds soften. Add spinach, kale, garlic, salt, and pepper to Instant Pot®.

3 Sauté for 4–6 minutes until greens begin to wilt. Press the Cancel button. Place greens in bowl for serving. Peel eggs, cut in half, and add to bowl. Slice avocado and place in bowl. Sprinkle red pepper flakes over all. Serve warm.

CALORIES: 649
PROTEIN: 21.3 grams
FIBER: 9.2 grams
NET CARBOHYDRATES: 6.0 grams

FAT: 55.2 grams
SODIUM: 1,336 milligrams
CARBOHYDRATES: 15.2 grams
SUGAR: 2.1 grams

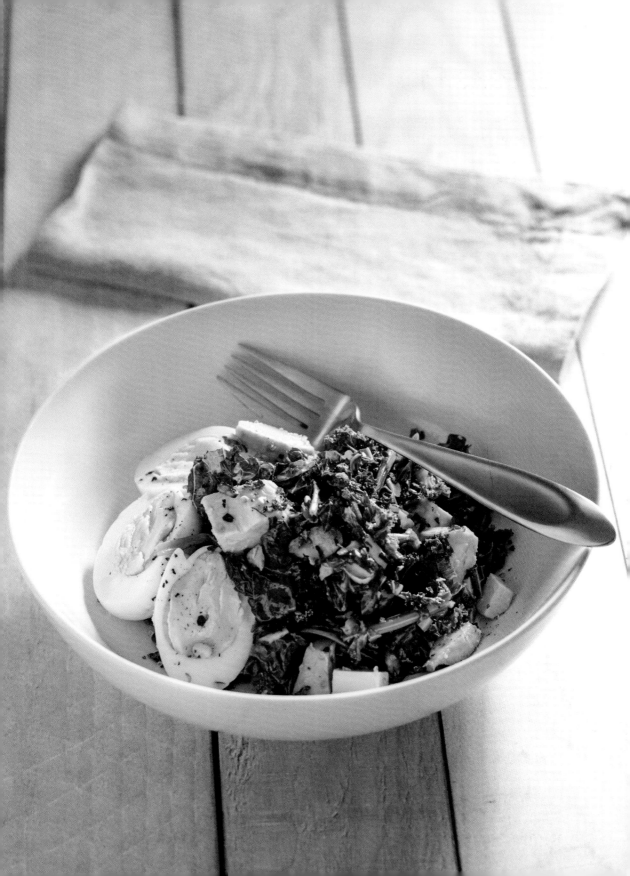

Poached Egg

There's nothing quite like yummy egg yolks with a savory breakfast dish. In just a few minutes and a fraction of the usual hassle, you can make a perfectly poached egg. Not a breakfast food lover? These are a great nutrient-rich addition to any burger!

- **Hands-on time:** 1 minute
- **Cook time:** 5 minutes

Serves 1

1 egg
1 cup water

1 Crack egg open into silicone baking cup. Pour water into Instant Pot®. Click lid closed.

2 Press the Manual button and adjust to Low Pressure. Set time for 5 minutes. When timer beeps, quick-release the pressure.

CALORIES: 71
PROTEIN: 6.3 grams
FIBER: 0.0 grams
NET CARBOHYDRATES: 0.4 grams

FAT: 4.3 grams
SODIUM: 62 milligrams
CARBOHYDRATES: 0.4 grams
SUGAR: 0.2 grams

Crispy Bacon

Bacon is a major keto staple and it's no secret why: it has zero carbs and tastes amazing! The downside of bacon is all the grease splatter. Cooking it in the Instant Pot® creates less splatter because of the pot's depth—and you don't have to sacrifice that delicious crunch!

- **Hands-on time:** 5 minutes
- **Cook time:** 10 minutes

Serves 2

4 slices bacon

1 Press the Sauté button and press the Adjust button to lower heat to Less. Add bacon to Instant Pot®. Allow it to fry for 5 minutes until it begins to render fat. Press the Cancel button.

2 Press the Sauté button and press the Adjust button to set heat to Normal. Continue frying bacon until desired crispness.

CALORIES: 107
PROTEIN: 7.8 grams
FIBER: 0.0 grams
NET CARBOHYDRATES: 0.4 grams

FAT: 7.7 grams
SODIUM: 387 milligrams
CARBOHYDRATES: 0.4 grams
SUGAR: 0.0 grams

Spaghetti Squash Fritters

Squash is super easy to cook in the Instant Pot® and has so many uses beyond just savory dinners. This dish is surprisingly flavorful and a breeze to make. Feel free to customize to your liking by adding your favorite filling items, such as mushrooms, chopped broccoli, or crumbled sausage.

- **Hands-on time: 20 minutes**
- **Cook time: 15 minutes**

Serves 4

½ cooked spaghetti squash
  (see Basic Spaghetti
  Squash in Chapter 5)
2 tablespoons cream cheese
½ cup shredded whole-milk
  mozzarella cheese
1 egg
½ teaspoon salt
¼ teaspoon pepper
1 stalk green onion, sliced
4 slices cooked bacon,
  crumbled
2 tablespoons coconut oil

KID FRIENDLY!

These are great to make for kids because they don't taste like squash. You get all the yummy bacon and onion flavor with much less of a veggie taste. It's a great way to sneak in some extra veggies! These can be served as the main dish or alongside a meal.

1 Remove seeds from cooked squash and use fork to scrape strands out of shell. Place strands into cheesecloth or kitchen towel and squeeze to remove as much excess moisture as possible.

2 Place cream cheese and mozzarella in small bowl and microwave for 45 seconds to melt together. Mix with spoon and place in large bowl. Add all ingredients except coconut oil to bowl. Mixture will be wet like batter.

3 Press the Sauté button and then press the Adjust button to set heat to Less. Add coconut oil to Instant Pot®. When fully preheated, add 2–3 tablespoons of batter to pot to make a fritter. Let fry until firm and completely cooked through.

CALORIES: 202
PROTEIN: 9.2 grams
FIBER: 0.3 grams
NET CARBOHYDRATES: 2.0 grams
FAT: 16.4 grams
SODIUM: 619 milligrams
CARBOHYDRATES: 2.3 grams
SUGAR: 0.9 grams

Breakfast Sausage Patties

Store-bought meat can be filled with preservatives and additives that make it last longer on the shelves. Instead, try flavoring your own breakfast sausage. It's a great feeling to avoid unnecessary ingredients and know exactly what is in your food. Feel free to add your favorite flavors. You can also cook these in advance and store (either cooked or uncooked) in the freezer between layers of parchment paper.

- **Hands-on time: 5 minutes**
- **Cook time: 15 minutes**

Serves 4

1 pound 84% lean ground pork
1 teaspoon dried thyme
½ teaspoon dried sage
½ teaspoon garlic powder
½ teaspoon salt
¼ teaspoon pepper
¼ teaspoon red pepper flakes

1 Mix all ingredients in large bowl. Form into 4 patties based on preference. Press the Sauté button and press the Adjust button to lower heat to Less.

2 Place patties in Instant Pot® and allow fat to render while patties begin browning. After 5 minutes, or when a few tablespoons of fat have rendered from meat, press the Cancel button.

3 Press the Sauté button and press the Adjust button to set heat to Normal. Sear each side of patties and allow them to cook fully until no pink remains in centers, approximately 10 additional minutes, depending on thickness.

CALORIES: 249	**FAT:** 15.5 grams
PROTEIN: 20.5 grams	**SODIUM:** 367 milligrams
FIBER: 0.2 grams	**CARBOHYDRATES:** 1.1 grams
NET CARBOHYDRATES: 0.9 grams	**SUGAR:** 0.0 grams

Mini Sausage Breakfast Bites

These sausage bites are so easy to prepare, pack, and pop on the go! We all have those hectic mornings when you have to get everyone up and out the door in a flash. This premade breakfast is a must-have for those days, and will give you the protein boost you need to keep you at your A-game!

- **Hands-on time:** 10 minutes
- **Cook time:** 15 minutes

Makes 32 balls; serving size 4 balls

---

1 pound breakfast sausage
1 ounce cream cheese, softened
1 egg
½ cup shredded sharp cheddar
1 cup water

MEAL PREP IT!

These are a great make-ahead item. If you want to freeze them, place cooked bites on a large cookie sheet and freeze for 1 hour. Then place in a freezer-safe storage bag. For a quick protein meal addition, reheat them in a skillet or microwave.

1 Mix all ingredients except water thoroughly and shape into round balls. Pour water into Instant Pot®. Place steam rack or Instant Pot®–safe bowl into pot and carefully put in sausage bites. Depending on your cooking vessel and pot size, this may require multiple batches. Click lid closed and adjust time for 15 minutes.

2 When timer beeps, quick-release pressure and remove meatballs. You may sear them on Sauté for a crunchy exterior or eat them as is. Serve warm.

CALORIES: 239
PROTEIN: 10.7 grams
FIBER: 0.0 grams
NET CARBOHYDRATES: 0.6 grams

FAT: 19.9 grams
SODIUM: 484 milligrams
CARBOHYDRATES: 0.6 grams
SUGAR: 0.1 grams

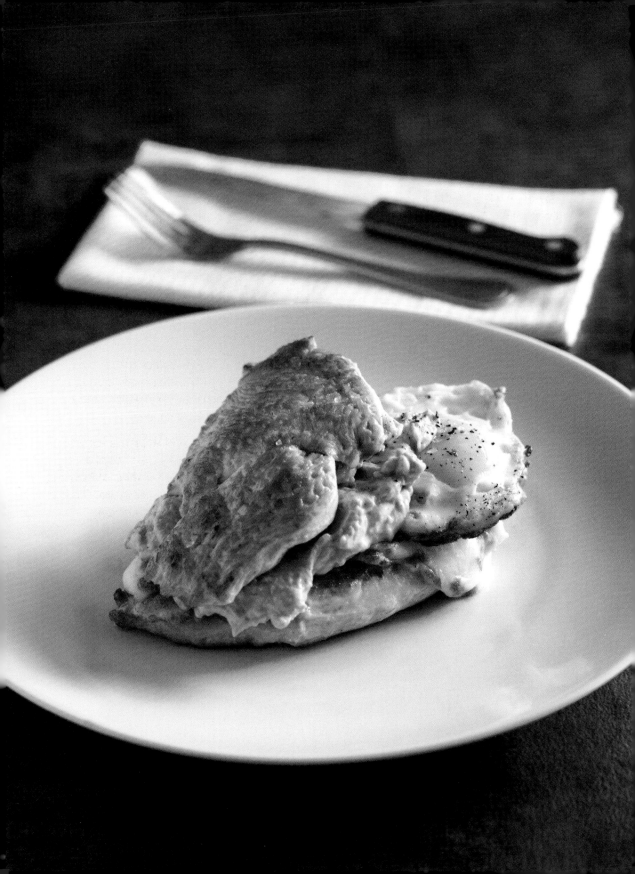

Chicken Breakfast Sandwich

Chicken is a unique yet wholesome way to start your day. This recipe makes chicken the star of a breakfast sandwich, replacing the bread you may be used to with chicken. It gives you a beneficial protein boost as part of a very fulfilling meal.

- **Hands-on time: 5 minutes**
- **Cook time: 15 minutes**

Serves 1

1 (6-ounce) boneless, skinless chicken breast
¼ teaspoon salt
⅛ teaspoon pepper
¼ teaspoon garlic powder
2 tablespoons coconut oil, divided
1 egg
1 cup water
¼ avocado
2 tablespoons mayo
¼ cup shredded white cheddar
Salt and pepper to taste

1 Cut chicken breast in half lengthwise. Use meat tenderizer to pound chicken breast until thin. Sprinkle with salt, pepper, and garlic powder, and set aside.

2 Add 1 tablespoon coconut oil to Instant Pot®. Press Sauté button, then press Adjust button and set temperature to Less. Once oil is hot, fry the egg, remove, and set aside. Press Cancel button. Press Sauté button, then press Adjust button to set temperature to Normal. Add second tablespoon of coconut oil to Instant Pot® and sear chicken on each side for 3–4 minutes until golden.

3 Press the Manual button and set time for 8 minutes. While chicken cooks, use fork to mash avocado and then mix in mayo. When timer beeps, quick-release the pressure. Put chicken on plate and pat dry with paper towel. Use chicken pieces to form a sandwich with egg, cheese, and avocado mayo. Season lightly with salt and pepper.

CALORIES: 761	**FAT:** 52.6 grams
PROTEIN: 52.4 grams	**SODIUM:** 996 milligrams
FIBER: 2.5 grams	**CARBOHYDRATES:** 5.2 grams
NET CARBOHYDRATES: 2.7 grams	**SUGAR:** 0.4 grams

Fried Egg and Avocado Sandwich

Does a sandwich need to have bread? Not anymore! Loading up on carbs in the morning can really bog you down and make you hungry earlier than you'd like. This speedy breakfast will fill you up with flavorful protein and lots of productivity-fueling fat. Trust me, you won't even miss the bread!

- **Hands-on time:** 5 minutes
- **Cook time:** 15 minutes

Serves 1

2 slices bacon
2 eggs
1 avocado

1 Press the Sauté button. Press the Adjust button to set heat to Low. Add bacon to Instant Pot® and cook until crispy. Remove and set aside.

2 Crack egg over Instant Pot® slowly, into bacon grease. Repeat with second egg. When edges become golden, after 2–3 minutes, flip. Press the Cancel button.

3 Cut avocado in half and scoop out half without seed. Place in small bowl and mash with fork. Spread on one egg. Place bacon on top and top with second egg. Let cool 5 minutes before eating.

CALORIES: 489
PROTEIN: 20.9 grams
FIBER: 4.6 grams
NET CARBOHYDRATES: 2.7 grams

FAT: 38.8 grams
SODIUM: 672 milligrams
CARBOHYDRATES: 7.3 grams
SUGAR: 1.1 grams

Get Up and Go Tea

Did you know many cold medicines are loaded with sugar? For a more natural cold remedy, this bold tea does the trick. The ginger is a bit spicy which helps clear out the sinuses and the apple cider vinegar provides the body with some great gut treatment to get you up and on your way.

- **Hands-on time: 5 minutes**
- **Cook time: 10 minutes**

Serves 1

1-inch section ginger root, sliced

1 tablespoon apple cider vinegar

½ lemon

2 cups water

Place ginger root into Instant Pot® with other ingredients. Press Sauté button and adjust temperature to Less. Let boil for 10 minutes. Strain and pour into cup to serve.

CALORIES: 4		**FAT:** 0.0 grams	
PROTEIN: 0.0 grams		**SODIUM:** 0 milligrams	
FIBER: 0.0 grams		**CARBOHYDRATES:** 0.5 grams	
NET CARBOHYDRATES: 0.5 grams		**SUGAR:** 0.1 grams	

Scrambled Eggs

The Instant Pot® brings convenience to your kitchen—it even makes scrambled eggs easier! You can even make scrambled eggs without turning on your stovetop. This traditional breakfast can be cooked up in no time and has a secret ingredient to make your eggs extra creamy.

- **Hands-on time: 5 minutes**
- **Cook time: 7 minutes**

Serves 4

6 eggs

2 tablespoons heavy cream

1 teaspoon salt

¼ teaspoon pepper

2 tablespoons butter

2 ounces cream cheese, softened

1 In large bowl, whisk eggs, heavy cream, salt, and pepper. Press the Sauté button and then press the Adjust button to set heat to Less.

2 Gently push eggs around pot with rubber spatula. When they begin to firm up, add butter and softened cream cheese. Continue stirring slowly in a figure-8 pattern until eggs are fully cooked, approximately 7 minutes total.

CALORIES: 232		**FAT:** 18.7 grams	
PROTEIN: 10.5 grams		**SODIUM:** 742 milligrams	
FIBER: 0.0 grams		**CARBOHYDRATES:** 1.4 grams	
NET CARBOHYDRATES: 1.4 grams		**SUGAR:** 1.0 grams	

Mini Maple Cake

Almond flour is a great alternative to traditional flour. It has only about a quarter of the carbs and many brands, such as Bob's Red Mill Super-Fine Almond Flour, do not have an overly nutty flavor. It does have its quirks and cooks differently than wheat flours, but you'll quickly learn the ins and outs and your body will thank you.

- **Hands-on time: 5 minutes**
- **Cook time: 20 minutes**

Serves 1

1 cup water
¼ cup almond flour
⅓ cup unsweetened almond milk
2 tablespoons coconut flour
1 egg
2 tablespoons erythritol
½ teaspoon vanilla extract
½ teaspoon maple extract
1 tablespoon melted butter

1 Pour water into Instant Pot®. In medium bowl, mix remaining ingredients. Pour into 4-inch ramekin or oven-safe mug. Cover with foil.

2 Place steam rack into pot and place mug on top. Click lid closed. Press the Manual button and adjust time for 20 minutes. When timer beeps, allow a natural release.

CALORIES: 392	FAT: 28.9 grams
PROTEIN: 8.7 grams	SODIUM: 155 milligrams
FIBER: 8.0 grams	CARBOHYDRATES: 38.9 grams
NET CARBOHYDRATES: 6.9 grams	SUGAR: 1.7 grams
SUGAR ALCOHOLS: 24.0 grams	

SUGAR ALTERNATIVES

Erythritol is a low-glycemic sugar alcohol that can be used as a sweetener. There are other low-glycemic sweeteners, such as stevia, that can be used also, depending on your personal preference. Be aware of high-glycemic sugar alcohols such as maltitol, which may spike your blood sugar.

Blackberry Cake

This is a good breakfast for fruit lovers who enjoy a little sweetness in the morning. Blackberries are one of the lowest glycemic berries, which make them an excellent choice for keto.

- **Hands-on time:** 10 minutes
- **Cook time:** 25 minutes

Serves 8

1 cup almond flour
2 eggs
½ cup erythritol
2 teaspoons vanilla extract
1 cup blackberries
4 tablespoons melted butter
¼ cup heavy cream
½ teaspoon baking powder
1 cup water

1 In large bowl, mix all ingredients except water. Pour into 7-inch round cake pan or divide into two 4-inch pans, if needed. Cover with foil.

2 Pour water into Instant Pot® and place steam rack in bottom. Place pan on steam rack and click lid closed. Press the Cake button and press the Adjust button to set heat to Less. Set time for 25 minutes.

3 When timer beeps, allow a 15-minute natural release then quick-release the remaining pressure. Let cool completely.

CALORIES: 174
PROTEIN: 9.8 grams
FIBER: 2.5 grams
NET CARBOHYDRATES: 2.7 grams
SUGAR ALCOHOLS: 12.0 grams
FAT: 14.6 grams
SODIUM: 51 milligrams
CARBOHYDRATES: 17.2 grams
SUGAR: 1.3 grams

Southwestern Frittata

Why not get your day started right with this savory and subtly spicy dish? If you aren't a fan of spicy flavors, a spoonful of sour cream on your plate will cool it down and add some extra fat to your meal.

- **Hands-on time: 5 minutes**
- **Cook time: 20 minutes**

Serves 4

2 tablespoons coconut oil
¼ cup diced onion
¼ cup diced green chilies
½ green bell pepper, diced
8 eggs
1 teaspoon salt
½ teaspoon chili powder
¼ teaspoon garlic powder
¼ teaspoon pepper
¼ cup heavy cream
4 tablespoons melted butter
½ cup shredded cheddar cheese
1 cup water
2 avocados
¼ cup sour cream

1 Press the Sauté button and add coconut oil to Instant Pot®. Add onion, chilies, and bell pepper. Sauté until onion is translucent and peppers begin to soften, approximately 3 minutes. While sautéing, whisk eggs, seasoning, heavy cream, and butter in large bowl. Pour into 7-inch round baking pan.

2 Press the Cancel button. Add onion and pepper mixture to egg mixture. Mix in cheddar. Cover pan with aluminum foil.

3 Pour water into Instant Pot®, and scrape bottom of pot if necessary to remove any stuck-on food. Place steam rack into pot and put in baking dish with eggs on top. Click lid closed.

4 Press the Manual button and set time for 25 minutes.

5 While food is cooking, cut avocados in half, remove pit, scoop out of shell and slice thinly. When timer beeps, quick-release the pressure. Serve with avocado slices and a spoonful of sour cream.

CALORIES: 563
PROTEIN: 18.4 grams
FIBER: 5.4 grams
NET CARBOHYDRATES: 4.8 grams

FAT: 47.1 grams
SODIUM: 877 milligrams
CARBOHYDRATES: 10.2 grams
SUGAR: 2.4 grams

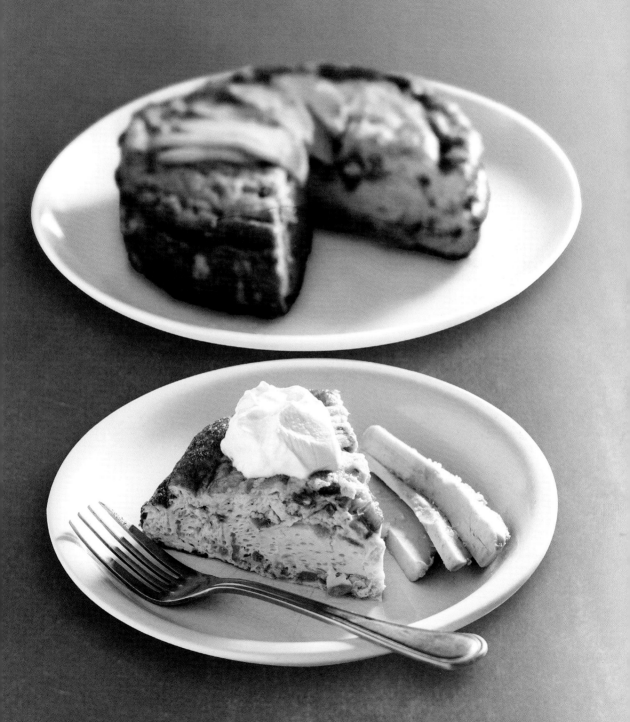

Sausage Pepper Gravy

For many people in the southern United States, breakfast time means sausage gravy. Traditionally made with flour, this gluten-free, keto-friendly alternative will wake you right up in the morning and have you reaching for a low-carb biscuit...or two!

- **Hands-on time: 5 minutes**
- **Cook time: 15 minutes**

Makes 2 cups; serving size ¼ cup

1 pound ground breakfast sausage
2 tablespoons butter
2 ounces cream cheese
1 cup heavy cream
½ teaspoon xanthan gum
½ teaspoon pepper
¼ teaspoon salt

1   Press the Sauté button and add breakfast sausage to Instant Pot®. Brown sausage until no pink remains, approximately 10 minutes. Add butter and cream cheese, stirring quickly until cream cheese is soft and smooth.

2   Press the Cancel button and add heavy cream. Continue stirring frequently as sauce begins to thicken. Add xanthan gum, pepper, and salt and stir until desired thickness, approximately 5–10 minutes. Serve warm with low-carb biscuits or eggs.

CALORIES: 316
PROTEIN: 9.8 grams
FIBER: 0.3 grams
NET CARBOHYDRATES: 1.7 grams

FAT: 27.7 grams
SODIUM: 530 milligrams
CARBOHYDRATES: 2.0 grams
SUGAR: 1.6 grams

MAKING LOW-CARB BISCUITS

There are lots of great recipes for keto-friendly biscuits online. Just be on the lookout for keto-friendly ingredients. Avoid wheat flours, honey, and generally milk in biscuit recipes. (Many keto biscuit recipes use mozzarella cheese or almond flour as a base.)

Vanilla Bean Custard

Need something on the sweeter side to coax you out of bed? This recipe is lightly sweet with aromatics that will brighten your morning. Even better, this breakfast is superfast so you'll have time to savor it even if you hit the snooze button a couple of times.

- **Hands-on time: 5 minutes**
- **Cook time: 7 minutes**

Serves 4

½ cup powdered erythritol
5 egg yolks
1 cup heavy cream
1 vanilla bean
1 cup water

DON'T WHIP IT!

To get a creamy texture, avoid using a whisk for this dish. Using a rubber spatula to combine the ingredients helps prevent air bubbles and gets you that creamy custard texture you're looking for.

1 In large bowl, use a rubber spatula to mix erythritol and egg yolks until smooth. (Do not use a whisk; it will add too much air to the mixture.)

2 Slowly pour in heavy cream while stirring gently until just combined. Scrape vanilla bean seeds into mixture and slowly combine.

3 Pour mixture into four (4-inch) ramekins and cover with foil. Pour water into Instant Pot® and place steam rack in pot. Place ramekins on steam rack. Click lid closed.

4 Press the Manual button and adjust time for 7 minutes. When timer beeps, allow a 10-minute natural release then quick-release the remaining pressure. Allow to cool completely uncovered then refrigerate, covered with plastic wrap, at least 2 hours.

CALORIES: 273
PROTEIN: 4.6 grams
FIBER: 9.0 grams
NET CARBOHYDRATES: 2.4 grams
SUGAR ALCOHOLS: 6.0 grams
FAT: 26.3 grams
SODIUM: 38 milligrams
CARBOHYDRATES: 17.4 grams
SUGAR: 7.8 grams

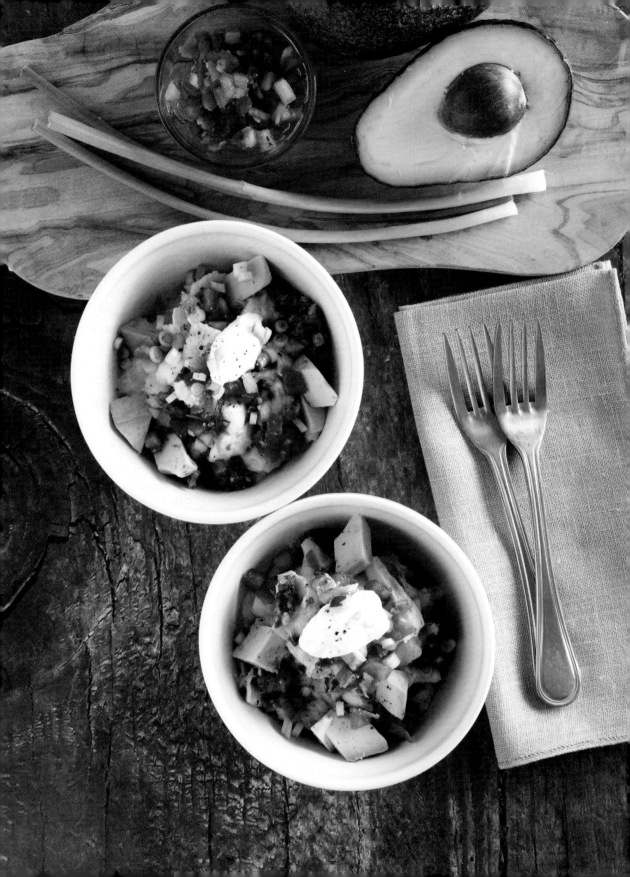

Breakfast Burrito Bowl

When you start a ketogenic diet, you will probably retrain what your brain thinks of in terms of food satisfaction. Empty calories like buns and tortillas aren't as appealing and certainly don't make the meal like they used to. Instead, you will have a greater appreciation for flavorful fillings like this bowl. It's full of fat to keep you full, even without a tortilla.

- **Hands-on time:** 10 minutes
- **Cook time:** 15 minutes

Serves 4

6 eggs

3 tablespoons melted butter

1 teaspoon salt

¼ teaspoon pepper

½ pound cooked breakfast sausage

½ cup shredded sharp cheddar cheese

½ cup salsa

½ cup sour cream

1 avocado, cubed

¼ cup diced green onion

1. In large bowl, mix eggs, melted butter, salt, and pepper. Press the Sauté button and then press the Adjust button to set the heat to Less.

2. Add eggs to Instant Pot® and cook for 5–7 minutes while gently moving with rubber spatula. When eggs begin to firm up, add cooked breakfast sausage and cheese and continue to cook until eggs are fully cooked. Press the Cancel button.

3. Divide eggs into four bowls and top with salsa, sour cream, avocado, and green onion.

CALORIES: 613

PROTEIN: 22.9 grams

FIBER: 4.0 grams

NET CARBOHYDRATES: 5.9 grams

FAT: 49.9 grams

SODIUM: 1,447 milligrams

CARBOHYDRATES: 9.9 grams

SUGAR: 1.6 grams

Sausage and Buffalo Egg Sandwich

Sometimes a little spice is just what you need to put some pep in your step. Some people love putting hot sauce on...well, everything, and eggs are no exception. This recipe replaces bread with two sausage patties and packs in lots of protein and healthy fats to keep you full and fueled.

- **Hands-on time:** 10 minutes
- **Cook time:** 15 minutes

Serves 1

2 uncooked breakfast sausage patties

1 egg

2 tablespoons cream cheese

2 tablespoons shredded sharp cheddar cheese

½ teaspoon hot sauce

¼ avocado, sliced

1 Press the Sauté button and add sausage patties to pot. Sear each side and continue cooking until no pink remains. Remove and set aside on a plate. Crack egg into hot Instant Pot® in leftover grease. Fry egg for approximately 3 minutes.

2 Press the Cancel button. Place egg onto one sausage patty. In small bowl, mix cream cheese, cheddar, and hot sauce. Microwave for 30 seconds and stir until smooth. Spread on second sausage patty. Place avocado slices on top of egg. Close sandwich by placing sausage patty on top of avocado.

CALORIES: 426
FAT: 32.6 grams
PROTEIN: 19.8 grams
SODIUM: 652 milligrams
FIBER: 2.3 grams
CARBOHYDRATES: 5.2 grams
NET CARBOHYDRATES: 2.9 grams
SUGAR: 1.7 grams

Soups and Chilis

Soups and chilis are ultimate comfort foods, especially when the weather is cool—even when the ingredients are keto-friendly. The meals in this chapter are hearty and nutritious and packed with tender meats, crisp veggies, and savory seasonings. Even better, the Instant Pot® cuts the cook time to a fraction of what you might expect on a stovetop or in a slow cooker. These soups and chilis are best served hot, but you can easily double (or triple) any of these recipes to freeze a portion for later. You'll be glad when the craving for Easy Jalapeño Popper Soup or White Chicken Chili hits and all you have to do is warm up what's already in your freezer!

Beef Broth

Beef Broth is an excellent base for soups and stews, and also a great go-to drink when you need a protein or sodium boost.

- **Hands-on time:** 5 minutes
- **Cook time:** 120 minutes

Makes 6 cups; serving size 1 cup

2 pounds beef bones
2 celery stalks, chopped
2 medium halved carrots
1 medium onion, peeled and halved
2 bay leaves
2 sprigs fresh thyme
6 cups water

1 Add all ingredients to Instant Pot®. Click lid closed. Press the Manual button and adjust time for 120 minutes.

2 When timer beeps, allow a full natural release. When pressure valve drops, remove large pieces of vegetables. Pour broth through fine-mesh strainer and store in closed containers in fridge or freezer.

CALORIES: 23
PROTEIN: 1.4 grams
FIBER: 0.1 grams
NET CARBOHYDRATES: 0.4 grams
FAT: 1.6 grams
SODIUM: 6 milligrams
CARBOHYDRATES: 0.5 grams
SUGAR: 0.2 grams

Chicken Broth

Homemade chicken broth is not only easy, but much more delicious than store-bought broth. As an added bonus, you can control the sodium amount to your liking. Next time you make a whole chicken, save the bones and use them for this basic broth.

- **Hands-on time:** 5 minutes
- **Cook time:** 120 minutes

Makes 6 cups; serving size 1 cup

2 pounds chicken bones
2 celery stalks, chopped
2 medium halved carrots
1 medium onion, peeled and halved
2 bay leaves
2 sprigs fresh thyme
6 cups water

1 Add all ingredients to Instant Pot®. Click lid closed. Press the Manual button and adjust time for 120 minutes.

2 When timer beeps, allow a full natural release. When pressure valve drops, remove large pieces of vegetables. Pour broth through fine-mesh strainer and store in closed containers in fridge or freezer.

CALORIES: 21
PROTEIN: 1.7 grams
FIBER: 0.1 grams
NET CARBOHYDRATES: 0.3 grams
FAT: 1.2 grams
SODIUM: 7 milligrams
CARBOHYDRATES: 0.4 grams
SUGAR: 0.2 grams

Bone Broth

This recipe will help you utilize every part of your chicken. The apple cider vinegar is the key ingredient in bone broth as it helps extract nutrients from the bones. The bones contain a wealth of proteins and minerals, and many low-carb followers drink the broth by itself to fill up on their anti-inflammatory, digestive, and joint-health benefits. Chicken bone broth also makes a great foundation for soups!

- **Hands-on time:** 5 minutes
- **Cook time:** 3 hours

Makes 6 cups; serving size 1 cup

2–3 pounds leftover chicken bones

3 tablespoons coconut oil

2 medium halved carrots

2 celery stalks, chopped

2 tablespoons apple cider vinegar

1 medium onion, large dice

2 whole cloves garlic

2 bay leaves

8 cups water

1 Press the Sauté button and add meat bones and coconut oil to Instant Pot®. Sauté for 5 minutes. Press the Cancel button.

2 Add remaining ingredients to pot and press the Soup button. Press the Adjust button to set heat to More. Set time for 3 hours. When timer beeps, allow a 20-minute natural release. Quick-release the remaining pressure.

3 Strain liquid and store in sealed jars in fridge up to 5 days.

CALORIES: 78
PROTEIN: 2.6
FIBER: 0.1 grams
NET CARBOHYDRATES: 0.4 grams

FAT: 6.9 grams
SODIUM: 13 milligrams
CARBOHYDRATES: 0.5 grams
SUGAR: 0.2 grams

BENEFITS OF BONE BROTH

Bone broth contains collagen, which helps hair, skin, and nails. It also has shown evidence to aid in joint healing and digestion.

Seafood Stock

Similar to other broths, Seafood Stock makes a great base for seafood recipes like gumbo and crab boils. Instead of immediately tossing your seafood shells, use them right away to make this stock, or freeze in a bag until you're ready.

- **Hands-on time:** 5 minutes
- **Cook time:** 120 minutes

Makes 6 cups; serving size 1 cup

4 cups shellfish shells
6 cups water
1 medium onion, peeled and chopped
2 tablespoons apple cider vinegar
2 bay leaves
2 celery stalks, chopped

1 Add all ingredients to Instant Pot®. Click lid closed. Press the Manual button and adjust time for 120 minutes.

2 Allow a 30-minute natural release, then quick-release the remaining pressure. When pressure valve drops, strain stock and store in sealed containers in fridge for 1–2 days or freeze.

CALORIES: 10
PROTEIN: 1.8 grams
FIBER: 0.1 grams
NET CARBOHYDRATES: 0.2 grams
FAT: 0.1 grams
SODIUM: 75 milligrams
CARBOHYDRATES: 0.3 grams
SUGAR: 0.1 grams

STORE IT FOR LATER
Seafood stock can be difficult to find in the grocery store, depending on where you live. Make and freeze this stock for when you need it for a flavorful boost to your seafood dishes.

Greek Lemon Soup

The simple ingredients in this traditional favorite create a creamy and light-tasting soup that's great for fighting colds. This recipe is perfect for using up leftovers, and you don't even need to use a pressure program for it.

- **Hands-on time: 5 minutes**
- **Cook time: 15 minutes**

Serves 4

4 cups Chicken Broth (see recipe in this chapter)
4 eggs, separated
1 lemon

MAKE THIS SOUP A MEAL

Whipping the egg whites makes this soup creamy without using dairy ingredients. Try adding chicken and cauliflower rice to this soup to make it more filling, or simply enjoy it as a broth to sooth a sore throat.

1 Press the Sauté button. Add Chicken Broth to Instant Pot® to warm.

2 In two medium bowls, separate egg yolks and egg whites. Beat egg yolks and stir into broth. Press the Cancel button so Instant Pot® switches to Stay Warm mode.

3 Using whisk or hand mixer, whisk egg whites until they form soft peaks. Add into Instant Pot®. Squeeze in juice from lemon. Foam may stay at the top of soup initially, but with continued occasional stirring, will dissipate by the end of cooking.

CALORIES: 93
PROTEIN: 7.9 grams
FIBER: 0.1 grams
NET CARBOHYDRATES: 1.2 grams

FAT: 5.5 grams
SODIUM: 77 milligrams
CARBOHYDRATES: 1.3 grams
SUGAR: 0.6 grams

Chicken Zoodle Soup

Whether you're looking to warm up on a chilly evening or to soothe a sore throat, this nutritious and hearty recipe for Chicken Zoodle Soup is exactly what you need. With a hint of spiciness to clear out the sinuses and a ton of veggies to nourish the body, this soup is just what the doctor ordered!

- **Hands-on time:** 15 minutes
- **Cook time:** 20 minutes

Serves 6

3 stalks celery, diced

2 tablespoons diced pickled jalapeño

1 cup bok choy, sliced into strips

½ cup fresh spinach

3 zucchini, spiralized

1 tablespoon coconut oil

¼ cup button mushrooms, diced

¼ medium onion, diced

2 cups cooked diced chicken

3 cups Chicken Broth (see recipe in this chapter)

1 bay leaf

1 teaspoon salt

½ teaspoon garlic powder

⅛ teaspoon cayenne pepper

COLD FIGHTER

This soup is a great alternative to chicken noodle and the cayenne kick is excellent for clearing out a stuffy head. A squeeze of lemon juice makes for a tasty addition with some vitamin C.

1 Place celery, jalapeño, bok choy, and spinach into medium bowl. Spiralize zucchini; set aside in a separate medium bowl. (The zucchini will not go in the pot during the pressure cooking.)

2 Press the Sauté button and add the coconut oil to Instant Pot®. Once the oil is hot, add mushrooms and onion. Sauté for 4–6 minutes until onion is translucent and fragrant. Add celery, jalapeños, bok choy, and spinach to Instant Pot®. Cook for additional 4 minutes. Press the Cancel button.

3 Add cooked diced chicken, broth, bay leaf, and seasoning to Instant Pot®. Click lid closed. Press the Soup button and set time for 20 minutes.

4 When timer beeps, allow a 10-minute natural release, and quick-release the remaining pressure. Add spiralized zucchini on Keep Warm mode and cook for additional 10 minutes or until tender. Serve warm.

CALORIES: 111	FAT: 3.7 grams
PROTEIN: 13.2 grams	SODIUM: 445 milligrams
FIBER: 1.7 grams	CARBOHYDRATES: 5.0 grams
NET CARBOHYDRATES: 3.3 grams	SUGAR: 3.3 grams

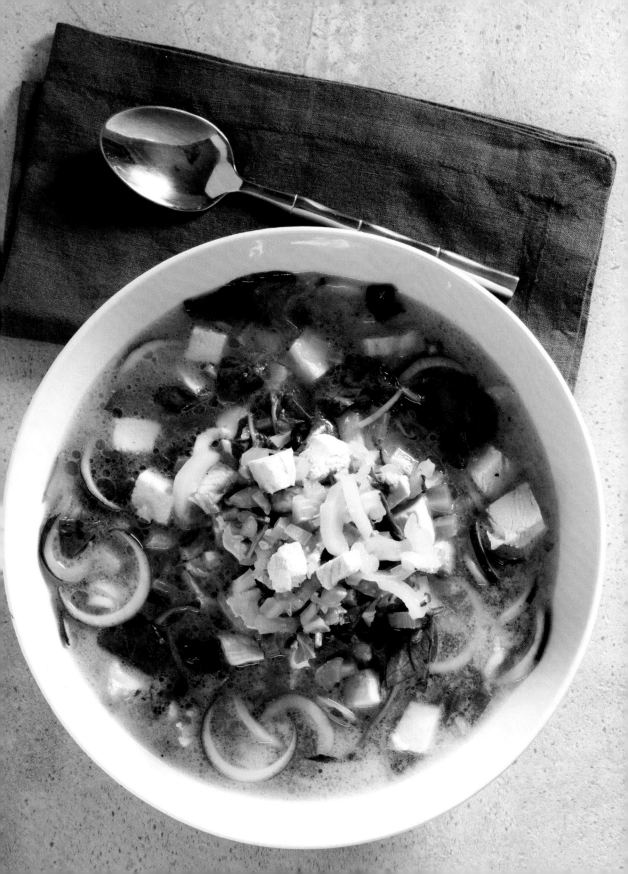

Beef Stew

This hearty dish is always a crowd-pleaser. It can be made using either the pressure cooking program or the slow cooker function. Feel free to add more veggies such as cauliflower to make this an even more filling dish—just be sure to add them toward the end of cooking so they don't overcook.

- **Hands-on time:** 15 minutes
- **Cook time:** 30 minutes

Serves 4

2 tablespoons coconut oil
1 pound cubed chuck roast
1 cup sliced button
    mushrooms
½ medium onion, chopped
2 cups Beef Broth (see
    recipe in this chapter)
½ cup chopped celery
1 tablespoon tomato paste
1 teaspoon thyme
2 garlic cloves, minced
½ teaspoon xanthan gum

WHY XANTHAN GUM?

Xanthan gum is a thickener that is often used in ketogenic cooking. It does not alter the flavor. If you don't mind a thinner soup, feel free to leave it out.

1 Press the Sauté button and add coconut oil to Instant Pot®. Brown cubes of chuck roast until golden, working in batches if necessary. (If the pan is overcrowded, they will not brown properly.) Set aside after browning is completed.

2 Add mushrooms and onions to pot. Sauté until mushrooms begin to brown and onions are translucent. Press the Cancel button.

3 Add broth to Instant Pot®. Use wooden spoon to scrape bits from bottom if necessary. Add celery, tomato paste, thyme, and garlic. Click lid closed. Press the Manual button and adjust time for 35 minutes. When timer beeps, allow a natural release.

4 When pressure valve drops, stir in xanthan gum and allow to thicken. Serve warm.

CALORIES: 354	**FAT:** 25 grams
PROTEIN: 23.6 grams	**SODIUM:** 89 milligrams
FIBER: 1.5 grams	**CARBOHYDRATES:** 4.4 grams
NET CARBOHYDRATES: 2.9 grams	**SUGAR:** 1.7 grams

Buffalo Chicken Soup

This recipe features a unique combination of spicy and creamy flavors. It's also an easier way to get those bold flavors from hot sauce without all the fuss of frying wings.

- **Hands-on time:** 5 minutes
- **Cook time:** 25 minutes

Serves 4

2 tablespoons diced onion

2 tablespoons butter

3 cups Chicken Broth (see recipe in this chapter)

2 (6-ounce) boneless, skinless chicken breasts, cubed

1 teaspoon salt

¼ teaspoon garlic powder

¼ teaspoon pepper

2 celery stalks, chopped

½ cup hot sauce

4 ounces cream cheese

½ cup shredded cheddar cheese

¼ teaspoon xanthan gum

1. Press the Sauté button and add onion and butter to Instant Pot®. Sauté 2–3 minutes until onions begin to soften. Press the Cancel button.

2. Add broth and chicken to Instant Pot®. Sprinkle salt, garlic powder, and pepper on chicken. Add celery and hot sauce and place cream cheese on top of chicken. Click lid closed.

3. Press the Manual button and adjust time for 25 minutes. When timer beeps, quick-release the pressure and stir in cheddar and xanthan gum. Serve warm.

CALORIES: 332

PROTEIN: 26.1 grams

FIBER: 1.0 grams

NET CARBOHYDRATES: 2.4 grams

FAT: 20.3 grams

SODIUM: 1,015 milligrams

CARBOHYDRATES: 3.4 grams

SUGAR: 1.6 grams

Garlic Chicken Soup

If you're a garlic lover, this soup is for you. It's creamy, buttery, and uses chicken thigh meat, which is highly flavorful. If you don't have time to cook the chicken, feel free to grab a rotisserie chicken at the store and make this even faster! Just add the cooked chicken after softening the onions.

- **Hands-on time:** 5 minutes
- **Cook time:** 20 minutes

Serves 6

10 roasted garlic cloves (see sidebar)
½ medium onion, diced
4 tablespoons butter
4 cups Chicken Broth (see recipe in this chapter)
½ teaspoon salt
¼ teaspoon pepper
1 teaspoon thyme
1 pound boneless, skinless chicken thighs, cubed
½ cup heavy cream
2 ounces cream cheese

1 In small bowl, mash roasted garlic into paste. Press the Sauté button and add garlic, onion, and butter to Instant Pot®. Sauté for 2–3 minutes until onion begins to soften. Press the Cancel button.

2 Add Chicken Broth, salt, pepper, thyme, and chicken to Instant Pot®. Click lid closed. Press the Manual button and adjust time for 20 minutes.

3 When timer beeps, quick-release the pressure. Stir in heavy cream and cream cheese until smooth. Serve warm.

CALORIES: 291

FAT: 21.1 grams

PROTEIN: 17.4 grams

SODIUM: 313 milligrams

FIBER: 0.4 grams

CARBOHYDRATES: 3.9 grams

NET CARBOHYDRATES: 3.5 grams

SUGAR: 1.4 grams

HOW TO ROAST GARLIC

Peel skin off garlic but leave the head itself together. Trim the top of the garlic to expose the cloves. Drizzle with 1 teaspoon avocado oil, wrap in foil, and bake in the oven at 400°F for 40 minutes.

Easy Jalapeño Popper Soup

This soup comes with plenty of heat and bold flavor. The only thing you'll need to worry about with this easy crowd-pleaser is how to get second helpings before it's all gone! If you prefer a milder flavor, simply reduce the number of jalapeños.

- **Hands-on time:** 5 minutes
- **Cook time:** 25 minutes

Serves 4

2 tablespoons butter

½ medium diced onion

¼ cup sliced pickled jalapeños

¼ cup cooked crumbled bacon

2 cups Chicken Broth (see recipe in this chapter)

2 cups cooked diced chicken

4 ounces cream cheese

1 teaspoon salt

½ teaspoon pepper

¼ teaspoon garlic powder

⅓ cup heavy cream

1 cup shredded sharp cheddar cheese

1 Press the Sauté button. Add butter, onion, and sliced jalapeños to Instant Pot®. Sauté for 5 minutes, until onions are translucent. Add bacon and press the Cancel button.

2 Add broth, cooked chicken, cream cheese, salt, pepper, and garlic to Instant Pot®. Click lid closed. Press the Soup button and adjust time for 20 minutes.

3 When timer beeps, quick-release the steam. Stir in heavy cream and cheddar. Continue stirring until cheese is fully melted. Serve warm.

CALORIES: 524

PROTEIN: 34.9 grams

FIBER: 0.8 grams

NET CARBOHYDRATES: 7.8 grams

FAT: 35.8 grams

SODIUM: 1,298 milligrams

CARBOHYDRATES: 8.6 grams

SUGAR: 6.2 grams

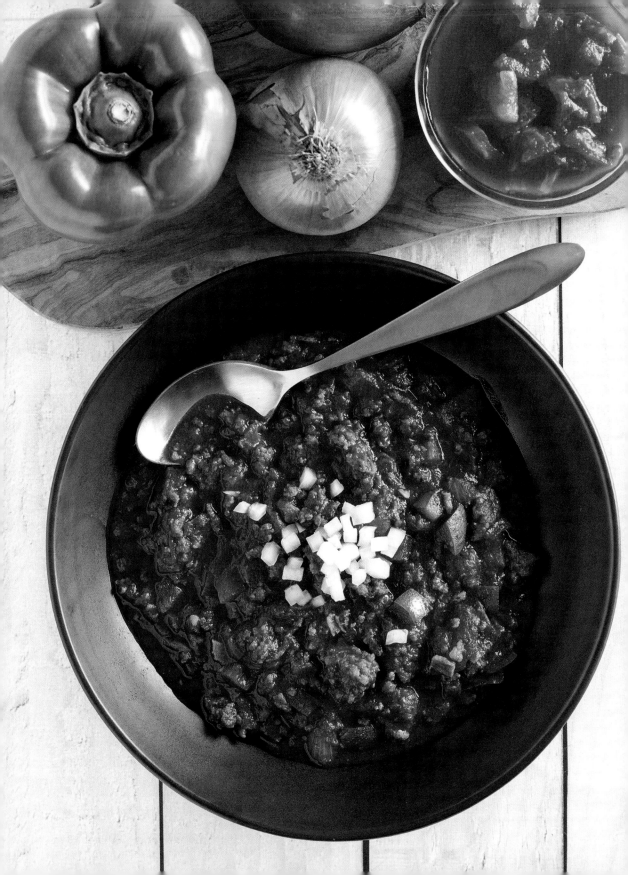

Red Chili

Eating a keto diet doesn't have to mean missing out on chili. Beans aren't even necessary to make this chili hearty and comforting. The flavor is packed into the broth, meat, and veggies that give it that classic chili taste without the carbs. This version packs a subtle punch of heat after the initial burst of flavor. Top with your favorite chili add-ins. For a crunch, try crushed pork rinds on top!

- **Hands-on time:** 10 minutes
- **Cook time:** 35 minutes

Serves 6

4 slices bacon
½ pound 85% lean ground beef
½ pound 84% lean ground pork
1 green pepper, diced
½ medium onion, diced
2 cups Beef Broth (see recipe in this chapter)
1 (14.5-ounce) can diced tomatoes
1 (6-ounce) can tomato paste
1 tablespoon chili powder
2 teaspoons salt
½ teaspoon pepper
⅛ teaspoon cayenne
¼ teaspoon xanthan gum (optional)

1 Press the Sauté button and cook bacon. Remove bacon and set aside. In bacon grease, brown beef and pork until fully cooked. Add green pepper and onion to Instant Pot®. Click lid closed.

2 Press the Cancel button and add remaining ingredients except xanthan gum to pot. Press the Soup button and adjust time for 30 minutes. Allow a 10-minute natural release and then quick-release the remaining pressure. Serve warm with favorite chili toppings.

3 For thicker chili, remove lid when timer goes off and press the Sauté button. Add xanthan gum and reduce chili, stirring frequently, until desired thickness. Top with additional diced onions or other toppings.

CALORIES: 294
PROTEIN: 18.9 grams
FIBER: 3.5 grams
NET CARBOHYDRATES: 8.7 grams
FAT: 17.7 grams
SODIUM: 1,135 grams
CARBOHYDRATES: 12.2 grams
SUGAR: 6.4 grams

Creamy Mushroom Soup

This soup is great by itself or can be used to help make casseroles and complement roasts. It's a great alternative to condensed soup meals, which often have many preservatives. To use it as a recipe enhancer rather than just a meal, simply reduce until thick and store in freezer or use immediately.

- **Hands-on time:** 10 minutes
- **Cook time:** 10 minutes

Serves 4

1 pound sliced button mushrooms

3 tablespoons butter

2 tablespoons diced onion

2 cloves garlic, minced

2 cups Chicken Broth (see recipe in this chapter)

½ teaspoon salt

¼ teaspoon pepper

½ cup heavy cream

¼ teaspoon xanthan gum

1 Press the Sauté button and then press the Adjust button to set heat to Less. Add mushrooms, butter, and onion to pot. Sauté for 5–8 minutes or until onions and mushrooms begin to brown. Add garlic and sauté until fragrant. Press the Cancel button.

2 Add broth, salt, and pepper. Click lid closed. Press the Manual button and adjust time for 3 minutes. When timer beeps, quick-release the pressure. Stir in heavy cream and xanthan gum. Allow a few minutes to thicken and serve warm.

CALORIES: 219
PROTEIN: 5.2 grams
FIBER: 1.6 grams
NET CARBOHYDRATES: 4.4 grams

FAT: 19.3 grams
SODIUM: 313 milligrams
CARBOHYDRATES: 6.0 grams
SUGAR: 3.4 grams

Cabbage Roll Soup

This soup is the perfect time-saver. Cabbage rolls are delicious but a bit tedious to make. With this recipe, you'll just toss everything in the pot and have this meal on the table in no time. It's a bit higher in carbs than some dishes as it has tomatoes, so be sure to plan it into your macros for the day.

- **Hands-on time:** 10 minutes
- **Cook time:** 8 minutes

Serves 4

- ½ pound 84% lean ground pork
- ½ pound 85% lean ground beef
- ½ medium onion, diced
- ½ medium head of cabbage, thinly sliced
- 2 tablespoons tomato paste
- ½ cup diced tomatoes
- 2 cups Chicken Broth (see recipe in this chapter)
- 1 teaspoon salt
- ½ teaspoon thyme
- ½ teaspoon garlic powder
- ¼ teaspoon pepper

1 Press the Sauté button and add beef and pork to Instant Pot®. Brown meat until no pink remains. Add onion and continue cooking until onions are fragrant and soft. Press the Cancel button.

2 Add remaining ingredients to Instant Pot®. Press the Manual button and adjust time for 8 minutes.

3 When timer beeps, allow a 15-minute natural release and then quick-release the remaining pressure. Serve warm.

CALORIES: 304	FAT: 15.6 grams
PROTEIN: 23.8 grams	SODIUM: 740 milligrams
FIBER: 4.1 grams	CARBOHYDRATES: 11.8 grams
NET CARBOHYDRATES: 7.7 grams	SUGAR: 6.1 grams

SLOW COOKER FRIENDLY!

If you prefer, you can make this meal using the slow cooker function as well. Brown meats, and then toss all the ingredients into the pot and use the slow cooker program on low for 8 hours (or high for 4 hours). Your home will smell delicious with a meal that's ready to eat.

Lobster Bisque

This classic dish is a smooth, richly seasoned soup loaded with juicy lobster. If you're not a fan of spicy foods, feel free to omit the cayenne.

- **Hands-on time:** 5 minutes
- **Cook time:** 10 minutes

Serves 4

4 tablespoons butter

½ medium onion, diced

1 clove garlic, finely minced

1 pound cooked lump lobster meat

½ teaspoon salt

¼ teaspoon pepper

¼ teaspoon paprika

⅛ teaspoon cayenne

2 tablespoons tomato paste

1 cup Seafood Stock (see recipe in this chapter)

1 cup Chicken Broth (see recipe in this chapter)

½ cup heavy cream

½ teaspoon xanthan gum

1　Press the Sauté button and add butter and onions to Instant Pot®. Sauté for 2–3 minutes until onions begin to soften. Add garlic and sauté 30 seconds. Press the Cancel button.

2　Add lobster, seasonings, tomato paste, and broths. Press the Manual button and adjust time for 7 minutes. When timer beeps, quick-release the pressure. Stir in heavy cream and xanthan gum. Allow a few minutes to thicken. Serve warm.

CALORIES: 328
PROTEIN: 23.7 grams
FIBER: 1.3 grams
NET CARBOHYDRATES: 3.5 grams

FAT: 22.4 grams
SODIUM: 882 grams
CARBOHYDRATES: 4.8 grams
SUGAR: 2.5 grams

DID YOU KNOW?
You can steam a lobster in the Instant Pot®! If you prefer fresh lobster, feel free to steam it and then use the fresh meat in this recipe.

Spicy Bacon Cheeseburger Soup

This Bacon Cheeseburger Soup will be a weekly staple in your house, especially in the colder months! This burger that you slurp from a spoon is comforting, cheesy, and doesn't miss a single flavor from the classic handheld version.

- **Hands-on time: 5 minutes**
- **Cook time: 15 minutes**

Serves 6

1 pound 85% lean ground beef

½ medium onion, sliced

½ (14.5-ounce) can fire-roasted tomatoes

3 cups Beef Broth (see recipe in this chapter)

¼ cup cooked crumbled bacon

1 tablespoon chopped pickled jalapeños

1 teaspoon salt

½ teaspoon pepper

½ teaspoon garlic powder

2 teaspoons Worcestershire sauce

4 ounces cream cheese

1 cup sharp cheddar cheese

1 pickle spear, diced

1 Press the Sauté button and add ground beef. Brown beef halfway and add onion. Continue cooking beef until no pink remains. Press the Cancel button. Add tomatoes, broth, bacon, jalapeños, salt, pepper, garlic powder, and Worcestershire sauce, and stir. Place cream cheese on top in middle.

2 Click lid closed. Press the Soup button and adjust time for 15 minutes. When timer beeps, quick-release the pressure. Top with diced pickles. Feel free to add additional cheese and bacon.

CALORIES: 358

PROTEIN: 23.5 grams

FIBER: 1.0 grams

NET CARBOHYDRATES: 4.6 grams

FAT: 24.0 grams

SODIUM: 908 milligrams

CARBOHYDRATES: 5.6 grams

SUGAR: 3.0 grams

KICK THE SPICE

If you're not a fan of spicy foods, simply omit the jalapeños from this dish. Feel free to add your personal favorite burger toppings to this—get creative!

Chicken and Cauliflower Rice Soup

This is a creamy and comforting soup that is perfect for a cold day inside. The veggies make this soup nutrient-rich and very filling.

- **Hands-on time:** 5 minutes
- **Cook time:** 20 minutes

Makes 4 cups; serving size 1 cup

---

4 tablespoons butter

¼ cup diced onion

2 stalks celery, chopped

½ cup fresh spinach

½ teaspoon salt

¼ teaspoon pepper

¼ teaspoon dried thyme

¼ teaspoon dried parsley

1 bay leaf

2 cups Chicken Broth (see recipe in this chapter)

2 cups diced cooked chicken

¾ cup uncooked cauliflower rice

½ teaspoon xanthan gum (optional)

1 Press the Sauté button and add butter to Instant Pot®. Add onions and sauté until translucent. Place celery and spinach into Instant Pot® and sauté for 2–3 minutes until spinach is wilted. Press the Cancel button.

2 Sprinkle seasoning into Instant Pot® and add bay leaf, broth, and cooked chicken. Click lid closed. Press the Soup button and adjust time for 10 minutes.

3 When timer beeps, quick-release the pressure and stir in cauliflower rice. Leave Instant Pot® on Keep Warm setting to finish cooking cauliflower rice additional 10 minutes. Serve warm.

4 For a thicker soup, stir in xanthan gum.

CALORIES: 228

PROTEIN: 22.4 grams

FIBER: 1.5 grams

NET CARBOHYDRATES: 1.5 grams

FAT: 13.7 grams

SODIUM: 471 grams

CARBOHYDRATES: 3.0 grams

SUGAR: 1.1 grams

Broccoli Cheddar Soup

Fill your home with the distinct aroma—and your mouth with the classic taste—of this low-carb Broccoli Cheddar Soup. Skip the restaurant versions and make this even better one at home. Want to bring this delicious autumn dish to the next level? Add crumbled bacon on top before serving.

- **Hands-on time: 5 minutes**
- **Cook time: 10 minutes**

Serves 4

2 tablespoons butter

⅛ cup onion, diced

½ teaspoon garlic powder

½ teaspoon salt

¼ teaspoon pepper

2 cups Chicken Broth (see recipe in this chapter)

1 cup broccoli, chopped

¼ cup heavy cream

1 tablespoon cream cheese, softened

1 cup shredded cheddar cheese

1 Press the Sauté button and add butter to Instant Pot®. Add onion and sauté until translucent. Press the Cancel button and add garlic powder, salt, pepper, broth, and broccoli to pot.

2 Click lid closed. Press the Soup button and set time for 5 minutes. When timer beeps, stir in heavy cream, cream cheese, and cheddar.

CALORIES: 249	**FAT:** 20.5 grams
PROTEIN: 9.0 grams	**SODIUM:** 357 milligrams
FIBER: 0.8 grams	**CARBOHYDRATES:** 3.5 grams
NET CARBOHYDRATES: 2.7 grams	**SUGAR:** 1.3 grams

Creamy Tuscan Soup

Soup is traditionally a cold-weather favorite, but don't forget about it in hotter months! This soup is creamy, but light enough to enjoy even on the hottest day. The fresh ingredients combined with a creamy sauce make a savory soup filled with nutrients.

- **Hands-on time:** 5 minutes
- **Cook time:** 17 minutes

Serves 4

4 slices bacon

1 pound ground Italian sausage

4 tablespoons butter

½ medium onion, diced

2 cloves garlic, finely minced

3 cups Chicken Broth (see recipe in this chapter)

4 ounces cream cheese

2 cups kale, chopped

½ cup heavy cream

1 teaspoon salt

½ teaspoon pepper

1. Press the Sauté button and fry bacon until crispy. Remove bacon and chop into pieces, then set aside. Add Italian sausage to Instant Pot® and sauté until no pink remains.

2. Add butter and onion to Instant Pot®. Sauté until onions are translucent. Add garlic and sauté for 30 seconds. Press the Cancel button.

3. Add broth and cream cheese to pot. Click lid closed. Press the Soup button and adjust time for 7 minutes.

4. When timer beeps, quick-release the pressure and add remaining ingredients to pot. Leave Instant Pot® on Keep Warm setting and allow to cook additional 10 minutes, stirring occasionally until kale is wilted. Serve warm.

CALORIES: 836

PROTEIN: 23.9 grams

FIBER: 0.7 grams

NET CARBOHYDRATES: 5.3 grams

FAT: 74.4 grams

SODIUM: 1,720 milligrams

CARBOHYDRATES: 6.0 grams

SUGAR: 3.0 grams

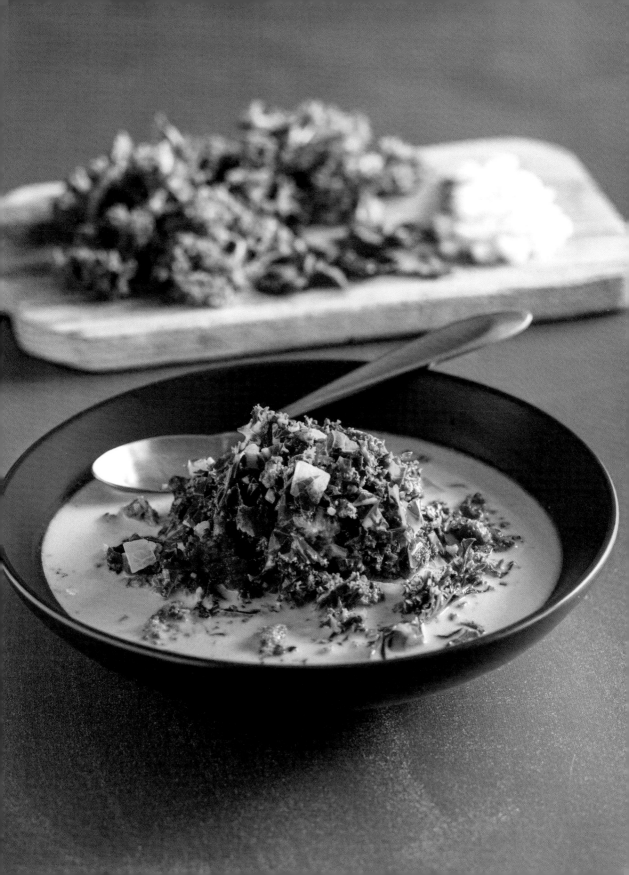

Chicken Bacon Chowder

Bacon makes everything better. This soup is loaded with bacon—and veggies for balance. It has plenty of healthy fat so it will help you stay full all day. A big leafy green salad would make an excellent companion to this dish.

- **Hands-on time:** 10 minutes
- **Cook time:** 20 minutes

Serves 6

½ pound bacon

1 teaspoon salt

½ teaspoon pepper

½ teaspoon garlic powder

¼ teaspoon dried thyme

3 (6-ounce) boneless, skinless chicken breasts

½ cup button mushrooms, sliced

½ medium onion, diced

1 cup broccoli florets

½ cup cauliflower florets

4 ounces cream cheese

3 cups Chicken Broth (see recipe in this chapter)

½ cup heavy cream

1 Press the Sauté button and then press the Adjust button to lower heat to Less. Add bacon to Instant Pot® and fry for a few minutes until fat begins to render, working in multiple batches if necessary. Press the Cancel button.

2 Press the Sauté button and then press the Adjust button to set heat to Normal. Continue frying bacon until fully cooked and crispy. Remove from pot and set aside. Sprinkle salt, pepper, garlic powder, and thyme over chicken breasts. Sear each side of the chicken for 3–5 minutes or until dark and golden. Press the Cancel button.

3 Add mushrooms, onion, broccoli, cauliflower, cream cheese, and broth to pot with chicken. Click lid closed. Press the Manual button and adjust time for 12 minutes. When timer beeps, quick-release the pressure. Remove chicken and shred or dice; add to pot. Crumble cooked bacon and stir into pot with heavy cream. Serve warm.

CALORIES: 407

PROTEIN: 26.5 grams

FIBER: 0.9 grams

NET CARBOHYDRATES: 3.8 grams

FAT: 28.1 grams

SODIUM: 760 milligrams

CARBOHYDRATES: 4.7 grams

SUGAR: 2.5 grams

White Chicken Chili

It's easy to cook this flavorful chili and even easier to make a double batch so you have some for the freezer! Whether you're pressure cooking or letting it slow cook all day, it's sure to be a hit. The tender chicken mixed with the peppers and cream cheese makes for a creamy and filling dish. Top with your favorite additions, like shredded cheese, diced jalapeños, sour cream, avocado—or all four!

- **Hands-on time:** 15 minutes
- **Cook time:** 20 minutes

Serves 6

4 tablespoons butter

¼ cup chopped onions

1 (4-ounce) can green chilies, drained

2 cloves garlic, minced

1 green pepper, chopped

1½ cups Chicken Broth (see recipe in this chapter)

1 pound boneless, skinless chicken breasts, cubed

1 teaspoon salt

¼ teaspoon pepper

4 ounces cream cheese

¼ cup heavy cream

1 Press the Sauté button and place butter and onions into Instant Pot®. Sauté until onions are fragrant and translucent. Add chilies, garlic, and green pepper. Sauté for 3 minutes, stirring frequently.

2 Press the Cancel button and add broth, chicken, seasoning, and cream cheese to pot. Press the Manual button and adjust time for 30 minutes.

3 When timer beeps allow a 10-minute natural release and quick-release the remaining pressure. Stir in heavy cream.

CALORIES: 274	FAT: 17.5 grams
PROTEIN: 19.6 grams	SODIUM: 697 milligrams
FIBER: 1.1 grams	CARBOHYDRATES: 4.5 grams
NET CARBOHYDRATES: 3.4 grams	SUGAR: 2.4 grams

TOP IT WITH AVOCADO!

Avocado is a keto superfood. It has a lot of fiber, so the net carbs are low but fat content is high, meaning it will help keep you full. Avocados are also loaded with a ton of vitamins to improve overall health.

Chicken Cordon Bleu Soup

Cut the carbs by making this classic dish into a keto-friendly soup! This recipe can be a weeknight dinner that comes together in under 20 minutes. It's simple yet flavorful and would pair wonderfully with low-carb rolls.

- **Hands-on time:** 5 minutes
- **Cook time:** 15 minutes

Serves 6

2 (6-ounce) boneless, skinless chicken breasts, cubed

4 cups Chicken Broth (see recipe in this chapter)

½ cup cubed ham

8 ounces cream cheese

1 teaspoon salt

½ teaspoon pepper

½ teaspoon garlic powder

½ cup heavy cream

2 cups grated Swiss cheese

2 teaspoons Dijon mustard

1 Place all ingredients except heavy cream, cream cheese, and mustard into Instant Pot®. Click lid closed.

2 Press the Soup button and adjust time for 15 minutes. When timer beeps, quick-release the pressure. Stir in heavy cream, cheese, and mustard. Serve warm.

CALORIES: 439	FAT: 30.2 grams
PROTEIN: 28.9 grams	SODIUM: 791 milligrams
FIBER: 0.1 grams	CARBOHYDRATES: 4.8 grams
NET CARBOHYDRATES: 4.7 grams	SUGAR: 2.4 grams

Creamy Enchilada Soup

Spicy, creamy, and filling, this soup is all the things you want in a quick weeknight dinner. The ingredients are simple, but when combined, they become a flavor-packed dish. You will find more carbs in this dish because of the enchilada sauce, so make sure you plan your macros for the day.

- **Hands-on time:** 10 minutes
- **Cook time:** 40 minutes

Serves 6

2 (6-ounce) boneless, skinless chicken breasts
½ tablespoon chili powder
½ teaspoon salt
½ teaspoon garlic powder
¼ teaspoon pepper
½ cup red enchilada sauce
½ medium onion, diced
1 (4-ounce) can green chilies
2 cups Chicken Broth (see recipe in this chapter)
⅛ cup pickled jalapeños
4 ounces cream cheese
1 cup uncooked cauliflower rice
1 avocado, diced
1 cup shredded mild cheddar cheese
½ cup sour cream

1 Sprinkle seasoning over chicken breasts and set aside. Pour enchilada sauce into Instant Pot® and place chicken on top.

2 Add onion, chilies, broth, and jalapeños to the pot, then place cream cheese on top of chicken breasts. Click lid closed. Adjust time for 25 minutes. When timer beeps, quick-release the pressure and shred chicken with forks.

3 Mix soup together and add cauliflower rice, with pot on Keep Warm setting. Replace lid and let pot sit for 15 minutes, still on Keep Warm. This will cook cauliflower rice. Serve with avocado, cheddar, and sour cream.

CALORIES: 318	**FAT:** 18.9 grams
PROTEIN: 20.7 grams	**SODIUM:** 693 milligrams
FIBER: 3.3 grams	**CARBOHYDRATES:** 10.0 grams
NET CARBOHYDRATES: 6.7 grams	**SUGAR:** 5.4 grams

Loaded Taco Soup

Are your Taco Tuesdays getting boring? Give this recipe a try. Not every taco needs a tortilla, and this soup has all the flavor you're looking for without all the carbs. It can be topped with all your favorite mix-ins to create a unique flavor. It freezes well, so whip up a double batch!

- **Hands-on time:** 10 minutes
- **Cook time:** 10 minutes

Serves 4

1 pound 85% lean ground beef
½ medium onion, diced
1 (7-ounce) can diced tomatoes and chilies
1 teaspoon salt
1 tablespoon chili powder
2 teaspoons cumin
3 cups Beef Broth (see recipe in this chapter)
⅓ cup heavy cream
¼ teaspoon xanthan gum
1 avocado, diced
½ cup sour cream
1 cup shredded cheddar cheese
¼ cup chopped cilantro

1 Press the Sauté button and brown ground beef in Instant Pot®. When halfway done, add onion. Once beef is completely cooked, add diced tomatoes with chilies, seasoning, and broth.

2 Click lid closed. Press the Soup button and adjust time for 10 minutes. When timer beeps, quick-release the pressure. Stir in cream and xanthan gum. Serve warm and top with diced avocado, sour cream, cheddar, and cilantro.

CALORIES: 566	FAT: 40.9 grams
PROTEIN: 31.6 grams	SODIUM: 1,016 milligrams
FIBER: 4.5 grams	CARBOHYDRATES: 10.6 grams
NET CARBOHYDRATES: 6.1 grams	SUGAR: 3.7 grams

Appetizers and Snacks

Have an upcoming game-day party, potluck get-together, or just need a quick bite to have on hand between meals? The recipes in this chapter will fit the bill. With savory classics like Spinach Artichoke Dip and Simple Meatballs alongside highly flavored dishes such as Blackened Chicken Bites and Ranch, you'll be ready to host the party of the year while staying on track with your goals!

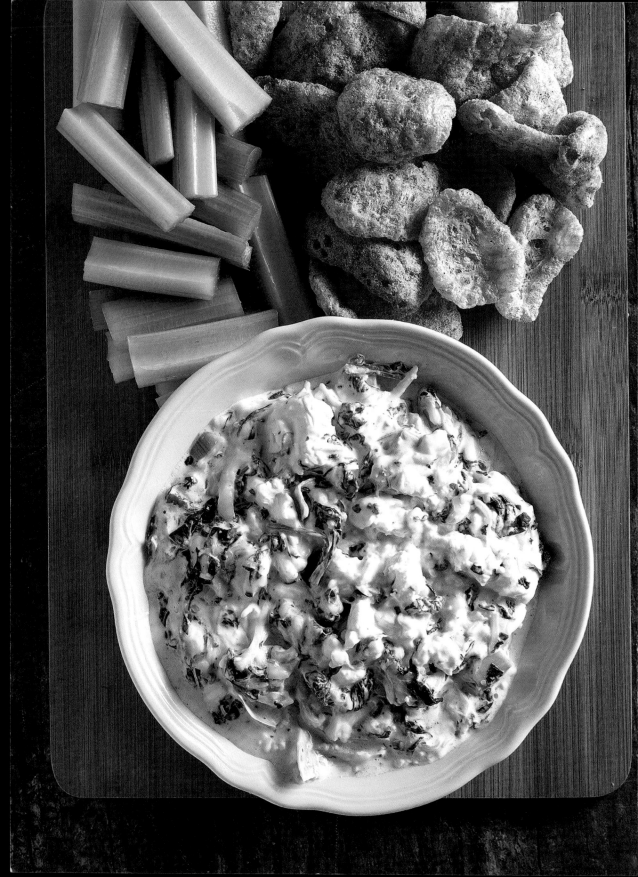

Spinach Artichoke Dip

This dip is always a favorite—and with good reason! It encourages sharing and casual chats. Skip the breadsticks or chips and instead enjoy with keto-friendly fresh veggie sticks and pork rinds.

- **Hands-on time:** 5 minutes
- **Cook time:** 7 minutes

Serves 6

½ cup Chicken Broth (see recipe in Chapter 3)

1 cup frozen spinach

½ cup sour cream

½ cup mayo

1 teaspoon garlic powder

½ teaspoon salt

1 (7-ounce) can artichokes, drained and chopped

8 ounces cream cheese

1½ cups shredded whole-milk mozzarella cheese

¼ cup grated Parmesan cheese

1 Pour broth into Instant Pot®. Add frozen spinach, sour cream, mayo, garlic, salt, and artichokes to Instant Pot®. Place cream cheese in pot.

2 Click lid closed. Press the Manual button and adjust time for 7 minutes. When timer beeps, quick-release the pressure.

3 Once valve drops down, open lid. Stir in mozzarella and Parmesan cheese. Serve warm.

CALORIES: 432
PROTEIN: 11.7 grams
FIBER: 1.3 grams
NET CARBOHYDRATES: 7.1 grams

FAT: 36.09 grams
SODIUM: 819 milligrams
CARBOHYDRATES: 8.4 grams
SUGAR: 2.5 grams

Bacon Chive Dip

Admit it, you've had dip that's so delicious you would eat it with a spoon. Well, get ready to add one more to your list of favorites! This delectable dip has enough pizzazz to elevate a family function all on its own! Enjoy with celery sticks.

- **Hands-on time:** 5 minutes
- **Cook time:** 10 minutes

Serves 6

1 pound bacon
8 ounces cream cheese
½ cup ranch dressing
½ cup sour cream
½ cup Chicken Broth (see recipe in Chapter 3)
1 cup shredded sharp cheddar cheese
¼ cup fresh chopped chives

1 Chop bacon into small pieces. Press the Sauté button. Press the Adjust button to set heat to Less. Add bacon to Instant Pot®. Once fat begins to render from bacon, after about 5 minutes, press the Cancel button.

2 Press the Sauté button and then press the Adjust button to set heat to Normal. Continue cooking bacon until crisp. When bacon is finished, remove and place on paper towel.

3 Press the Cancel button. Add cream cheese, ranch, sour cream, broth, and half of cooked bacon to pot and stir. Click lid closed. Press the Manual button and adjust time for 4 minutes.

4 When timer beeps, quick-release the pressure. When pressure valve drops, remove lid and stir. Add in remaining bacon, cheddar, and top with chives. Serve warm.

CALORIES: 564	**FAT:** 48.7 grams
PROTEIN: 16.9 grams	**SODIUM:** 780 milligrams
FIBER: 0.1 grams	**CARBOHYDRATES:** 3.5 grams
NET CARBOHYDRATES: 3.4 grams	**SUGAR:** 2.7 grams

Broccoli Cheddar Dip

This delicious and savory dip is like soup you can scoop! With ingredients similar to those in the soup version, but with added fat and thickness, this recipe is a wonderful dip for any weather and any time of year. Scoop it up with broccoli or cauliflower florets.

- **Hands-on time: 5 minutes**
- **Cook time: 10 minutes**

Serves 6

4 tablespoons butter

½ medium onion, diced

1½ cups chopped broccoli

8 ounces cream cheese

½ cup mayo

½ cup Chicken Broth (see recipe in Chapter 3)

1 cup shredded cheddar cheese

CHEESE IN THE INSTANT POT®

Cream cheese works well in long cooking programs, but shredded and cubed cheeses may stick to the pot, so it's best to leave them out of the pressure cooking program and stir them in at the end. Heavy cream is a popular ingredient in many ketogenic meals and will mix into soups and creamy sauces just fine after the pressure cooking program has ended.

1 Press the Sauté button and then press the Adjust button to set heat to Less. Add butter to Instant Pot®. Add onion and sauté until softened, about 5 minutes. Press the Cancel button.

2 Add broccoli, cream cheese, mayo, and broth to pot. Press the Manual button and adjust time for 4 minutes.

3 When timer beeps, quick-release the pressure and stir in cheddar. Serve warm.

CALORIES: 411

PROTEIN: 7.9 grams

FIBER: 0.8 grams

NET CARBOHYDRATES: 3.5 grams

FAT: 37.3 grams

SODIUM: 384 milligrams

CARBOHYDRATES: 4.3 grams

SUGAR: 2.2 grams

Hot Crab Dip

The irresistibly smooth and creamy texture combined with the perfect amount of crustaceous flavor will have you or your guests asking for more! Serve warm with veggies and pork rinds for scooping.

- **Hands-on time:** 5 minutes
- **Cook time:** 5 minutes

Serves 4

8 ounces cream cheese
1 pound cooked lump crab meat
¼ cup mayo
¼ cup sour cream
¼ teaspoon pepper
¼ teaspoon salt
½ tablespoon lemon juice
½ teaspoon hot sauce
¼ cup chopped pickled jalapeños
½ cup shredded cheddar
¼ cup chopped green onions
1 cup water

1 Place all ingredients in 7-cup glass bowl and mix. Cover with aluminum foil.

2 Pour water into Instant Pot® and place steam rack in bottom. Place bowl on steam rack and click lid closed. Press the Manual button and adjust time for 5 minutes. When timer beeps, quick-release the pressure. Stir.

CALORIES: 488
PROTEIN: 27.9 grams
FIBER: 0.6 grams
NET CARBOHYDRATES: 7.6 grams
FAT: 34.1 grams
SODIUM: 1,065 milligrams
CARBOHYDRATES: 8.2 grams
SUGAR: 6.6 grams

FRESH CRAB
This dip can also be made with fresh crab meat. Crab legs only take a few minutes to steam under pressure (see Snow Crab Legs with Butter Sauce recipe in Chapter 8).

Creamy Chorizo Dip

How can you go wrong with cheesy and spicy? You can't! This creamy dip packs the perfect kick, and it will keep you coming back for more. The great news is that with so few carbs, you can have just about as much as you want...guilt-free. Just keep your eye on what you eat it with—pork rinds are a great option.

- **Hands-on time:** 5 minutes
- **Cook time:** 10 minutes

Serves 4

1 pound ground chorizo
1 cup Chicken Broth (see recipe in Chapter 3)
½ cup salsa
8 ounces cream cheese
½ cup shredded white American cheese

1 Press the Sauté button and add chorizo to Instant Pot®. Cook thoroughly and drain or pat with paper towel to absorb grease.

2 Add broth and salsa. Place cream cheese on top of meat. Click lid closed. Press the Manual button to adjust time for 5 minutes.

3 When timer beeps, quick-release the pressure and stir in white American cheese. Serve warm.

CALORIES: 688
PROTEIN: 28.4 grams
FIBER: 0.4 grams
NET CARBOHYDRATES: 6.9 grams

FAT: 53.1 grams
SODIUM: 1,828 milligrams
CARBOHYDRATES: 7.3 grams
SUGAR: 2.7 grams

Buffalo Chicken Meatballs

A twist on a classic Swedish meatball appetizer, these meatballs are just as easy to make, but come with an exciting spicy kick. For an even bigger treat for your taste buds, finish off the recipe by garnishing your meatballs with blue cheese crumbles!

- **Hands-on time:** 5 minutes
- **Cook time:** 10 minutes

Serves 4

1 pound ground chicken
½ cup almond flour
2 tablespoons cream cheese
1 packet dry ranch dressing mix
½ teaspoon salt
¼ teaspoon pepper
¼ teaspoon garlic powder
1 cup water
2 tablespoons butter, melted
⅓ cup hot sauce
¼ cup crumbled feta cheese
¼ cup sliced green onion

1 In large bowl, mix ground chicken, almond flour, cream cheese, ranch, salt, pepper, and garlic powder. Roll mixture into 16 balls.

2 Place meatballs on steam rack and add 1 cup water to Instant Pot®. Click lid closed. Press the Meat button and set time for 10 minutes.

3 Combine butter and hot sauce. When timer beeps, remove meatballs and place in clean large bowl. Toss in hot sauce mixture. Top with sprinkled feta and green onions to serve.

CALORIES: 367
FAT: 24.9 grams
PROTEIN: 25.0 grams
SODIUM: 1,131 milligrams
FIBER: 1.8 grams
CARBOHYDRATES: 8.6 grams
NET CARBOHYDRATES: 6.8 grams
SUGAR: 1.3 grams

Buffalo Chicken Dip

A tangy flavor and rich, creamy texture make this recipe a go-to on game day. With so many low-carb dipping options from pork rinds to celery sticks, you'll have no trouble finding the bottom of this dip's bowl!

- **Hands-on time: 5 minutes**
- **Cook time: 20 minutes**

Serves 6

3 (6-ounce) boneless, skinless chicken breasts

1 teaspoon salt

½ teaspoon garlic powder

¼ teaspoon pepper

¾ cup Chicken Broth (see recipe in Chapter 3)

½ cup buffalo sauce

4 ounces cream cheese, softened

3 tablespoons butter

1 cup shredded cheddar cheese

1 Place chicken breasts in Instant Pot® and sprinkle both sides with salt, garlic powder, and pepper. Add broth and buffalo sauce to pot. Click lid closed and press the Manual button to adjust time for 20 minutes.

2 When timer beeps, allow a 5-minute natural release and then quick-release the remaining pressure. Shred chicken with two forks and mix in cream cheese, butter, and cheddar.

CALORIES: 297
PROTEIN: 25.1 grams
FIBER: 0.1 grams
NET CARBOHYDRATES: 1.2 grams

FAT: 20.4 grams
SODIUM: 1,230 milligrams
CARBOHYDRATES: 1.3 grams
SUGAR: 0.7 grams

Simple Meatballs

When it comes to classic appetizers, it doesn't get much simpler or more classic than these meatballs. These party favorites are rolled up and steamed, then simmered in a flavorful herb-filled tomato sauce. Don't forget to sprinkle them with Parmesan and oregano!

- **Hands-on time:** 5 minutes
- **Cook time:** 9 minutes

Serves 4

1 pound 85% lean ground beef
¼ cup almond flour
¼ cup grated Parmesan
1 egg
2 teaspoons dried parsley
1 teaspoon salt
½ teaspoon dried oregano
¼ teaspoon pepper
1 cup Easy Tomato Sauce (see recipe in this chapter)
½ cup Beef Broth (see recipe in Chapter 3)

1 In large bowl, mix ground beef, almond flour, Parmesan, egg, parsley, salt, oregano, and pepper. Fully combine and roll into 12 balls.

2 Place tomato sauce and broth in bottom of Instant Pot®. Add meatballs, turning each one to coat in sauce. Click lid closed. Press the Manual button and adjust time for 9 minutes.

3 When timer beeps, allow a 5-minute natural release and quick-release the remaining pressure. Spoon sauce over meatballs. Serve warm.

CALORIES: 326 grams
PROTEIN: 26.6 grams
FIBER: 2.4 grams
NET CARBOHYDRATES: 7.6 grams

FAT: 23.4 grams
SODIUM: 1,058 milligrams
CARBOHYDRATES: 10.0 grams
SUGAR: 4.5 grams

MAKE IT A MEAL
Although delicious by themselves, these meatballs can become a meal if you serve over buttery zucchini noodles and top with Parmesan cheese.

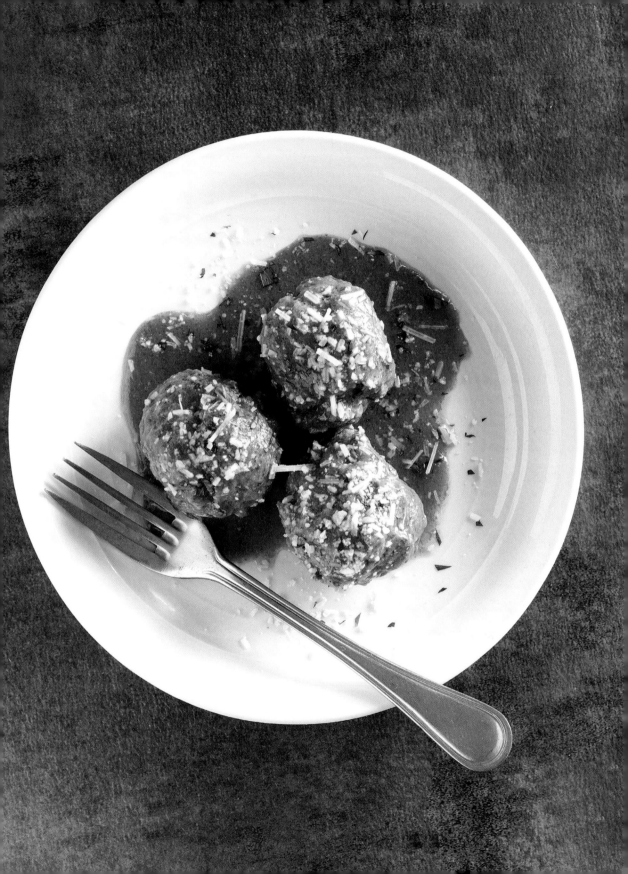

Tuna Deviled Eggs

If you love handy hacks to simplify complicated recipes, this appetizer will wow you! These aren't your mama's deviled eggs, but they are bursting with flavor. By filling the hard-boiled eggs with the tuna, seasoning, and veggies, in no time at all you'll have a bundle of bite-sized keto-friendly mini tuna salads!

- **Hands-on time:** 10 minutes
- **Cook time:** 8 minutes

Serves 3

1 cup water
6 eggs
1 (5-ounce) can tuna, drained
4 tablespoons mayo
1 teaspoon lemon juice
1 celery stalk, diced finely
¼ teaspoon Dijon mustard
¼ teaspoon chopped fresh dill
¼ teaspoon salt
⅛ teaspoon garlic powder

1. Add water to Instant Pot®. Place steam rack or steamer basket inside pot. Carefully put eggs into steamer basket. Click lid closed. Press the Egg button and adjust time for 8 minutes.

2. Add remaining ingredients to medium bowl and mix.

3. When timer beeps, quick-release the steam and remove eggs. Place in bowl of cool water for 10 minutes, then remove shells.

4. Cut eggs in half and remove hard-boiled yolks, setting whites aside. Place yolks in food processor and pulse until smooth, or mash with fork. Add yolks to bowl with tuna and mayo, mixing until smooth.

5. Spoon mixture into egg-white halves. Serve chilled.

CALORIES: 303
PROTEIN: 20.2 grams
FIBER: 0.2 grams
NET CARBOHYDRATES: 1.3 grams

FAT: 22.4 grams
SODIUM: 558 milligrams
CARBOHYDRATES: 1.5 grams
SUGAR: 0.7 grams

Avocado Egg Salad

If you've been enjoying a keto lifestyle for a while, you've more than likely paired avocados and eggs—two of your main pantry staples. Why? Because the healthy fats in the avocado keep you full and the protein in the eggs keep your muscles strong. This recipe marries the two foods for the perfect lunchtime dish. You can also add crunch to this recipe without putting on a single carb by topping it with bacon!

- **Hands-on time:** 10 minutes
- **Cook time:** 8 minutes

Serves 2

1 cup water
6 eggs
1 avocado
2 tablespoons lime juice
½ teaspoon chili powder
¼ teaspoon salt
2 tablespoons mayo
2 tablespoons chopped cilantro

1 Pour water into Instant Pot®. Place eggs on steam rack or in steamer basket inside pot.

2 Click lid closed. Press the Egg button and adjust time for 8 minutes. While egg is cooking, cut avocado in half and scoop out flesh. Place in food processor and blend until smooth.

3 Transfer avocado to medium bowl and add lime juice, chili powder, salt, mayo, and cilantro.

4 When timer beeps, carefully remove eggs and place in bowl of cold water for 5 minutes. Peel eggs and chop into bite-sized pieces. Fold chopped eggs into avocado mixture. Serve chilled.

CALORIES: 426
PROTEIN: 20.5 grams
FIBER: 5.0 grams
NET CARBOHYDRATES: 3.7 grams

FAT: 32.6 grams
SODIUM: 615 milligrams
CARBOHYDRATES: 8.7 grams
SUGAR: 1.2 grams

Chicken Spinach Meatballs

Getting tired of the classic meatball options? Try this keto-friendly kind that's light but filling. These cheesy meatballs make an excellent trifecta of flavor, protein, and fiber. Add them to your zoodles to make a spaghetti-like meal. If you're really in a hurry, they have more than enough flavor to eat by themselves!

- **Hands-on time:** 5 minutes
- **Cook time:** 15 minutes

Makes 12 meatballs; serving size 2 meatballs

1 pound ground chicken
½ cup frozen spinach
1 egg
½ cup shredded pepper jack cheese
1 ounce cream cheese
1 teaspoon salt
¼ teaspoon pepper
¼ teaspoon garlic powder
¼ teaspoon dried parsley
1 cup water
2 tablespoons coconut oil

1 Mix all ingredients except water and coconut oil in large mixing bowl. Roll into 12 balls. Pour water into Instant Pot® and place steamer rack in bottom. Place meatballs on rack. (You may have to cook in two batches.) Click lid closed.

2 Press the Manual button and adjust time for 10 minutes. When timer beeps, allow a 5-minute natural release. Quick-release the remaining pressure. Remove rack with meatballs and set aside. Pour out water and replace inner pot.

3 Press the Sauté button and add coconut oil to Instant Pot®. Once oil is heated, add meatballs until browned and crispy.

CALORIES: 216
PROTEIN: 17.3 grams
FIBER: 0.4 grams
NET CARBOHYDRATES: 0.8 grams
FAT: 14.9 grams
SODIUM: 528 milligrams
CARBOHYDRATES: 1.2 grams
SUGAR: 0.3 grams

Quick Queso

Queso is the king of appetizers. You simply can't have a gathering without it! This recipe is great for a late-night snack, or to bring to a game-day watch party. Excellent dippers would be pork rinds, cheese chips, and veggies, but you might just want to use a spoon!

- **Hands-on time:** 3 minutes
- **Cook time:** 10 minutes

Serves 6

8 ounces cream cheese, softened

½ cup sour cream

¼ cup heavy cream

2 tablespoons water

1 cup shredded Monterey jack cheese

1 cup shredded pepper jack cheese

1 cup cooked 85% lean ground beef mixed with ½ tablespoon taco seasoning

1 Press the Sauté button and add cream cheese, sour cream, heavy cream, and water Instant Pot®. Once mixture begins to boil, press the Cancel button.

2 Stir in remaining ingredients until smooth. Serve warm with pork rinds or veggies.

CALORIES: 404	**FAT:** 32.0 grams
PROTEIN: 18.1 grams	**SODIUM:** 448 milligrams
FIBER: 0.1 grams	**CARBOHYDRATES:** 3.4 grams
NET CARBOHYDRATES: 3.3 grams	**SUGAR:** 2.3 grams

PORK RINDS FOR DIPPING

Not sure what to dip? Pork rinds are a common low-carb chip replacement. They do have protein in them, so account for that in your day's nutrition. Sliced cucumbers and sliced celery also make great dippers.

Jalapeño Poppers

Spicy and creamy are always a great combo, and they're the central features of this crowd-pleasing appetizer. Bring these delightful poppers to your next potluck or family function, but make sure you grab some for yourself before you set them out...they'll be gone fast!

- **Hands-on time:** 10 minutes
- **Cook time:** 3 minutes

Serves 4

6 jalapeños
4 ounces cream cheese
¼ cup shredded sharp cheddar cheese
1 cup water
¼ cup cooked crumbled bacon

JALAPEÑOS AND SKIN IRRITATION

Jalapeños have oils that can cause skin irritation. You may want to wear gloves to cut them up to avoid contact with the oils.

1 Cut jalapeños lengthwise and scoop out seeds and membrane, then set aside.

2 In small bowl, mix cream cheese and cheddar. Spoon into emptied jalapeños. Pour water into Instant Pot® and place steamer basket in bottom.

3 Place stuffed jalapeños on steamer rack. Click lid closed. Press the Manual button and adjust time for 3 minutes. When timer beeps, quick-release the pressure. Serve topped with crumbled bacon.

CALORIES: 185	FAT: 14.3 grams
PROTEIN: 7.5 grams	SODIUM: 342 milligrams
FIBER: 0.6 grams	CARBOHYDRATES: 2.8 grams
NET CARBOHYDRATES: 2.2 grams	SUGAR: 1.8 grams

Easy Tomato Sauce

Tomato sauce is one staple every house should have on hand at all times. You can serve it warm over chicken or vegetable noodles, or with low-carb mozzarella sticks! Because store-bought jars of tomato sauce are often full of sugar, you'll want to make your own for your keto diet. This recipe will give you all of the savory goodness without the unnecessary carbs.

- **Hands-on time:** 5 minutes
- **Cook time:** 30 minutes

Makes 2½ cups; serving size ¼ cup

3 tablespoons butter
½ medium onion, finely diced
1 clove garlic, finely minced
2 (6-ounce) cans tomato paste
2 cups Chicken Broth (see recipe in Chapter 3)
1 teaspoon fresh parsley
½ teaspoon oregano
½ teaspoon basil

1 Press the Sauté button. Sauté onion until translucent. Add garlic and sauté for 30 seconds. Press the Cancel button.

2 Add remaining ingredients to Instant Pot® and stir. Click lid closed. Press the Manual button and adjust time for 30 minutes. When timer beeps, quick-release the pressure.

CALORIES: 65
PROTEIN: 1.9 grams
FIBER: 1.5 grams
NET CARBOHYDRATES: 5.7 grams

FAT: 3.6 grams
SODIUM: 270 milligrams
CARBOHYDRATES: 7.2 grams
SUGAR: 4.4 grams

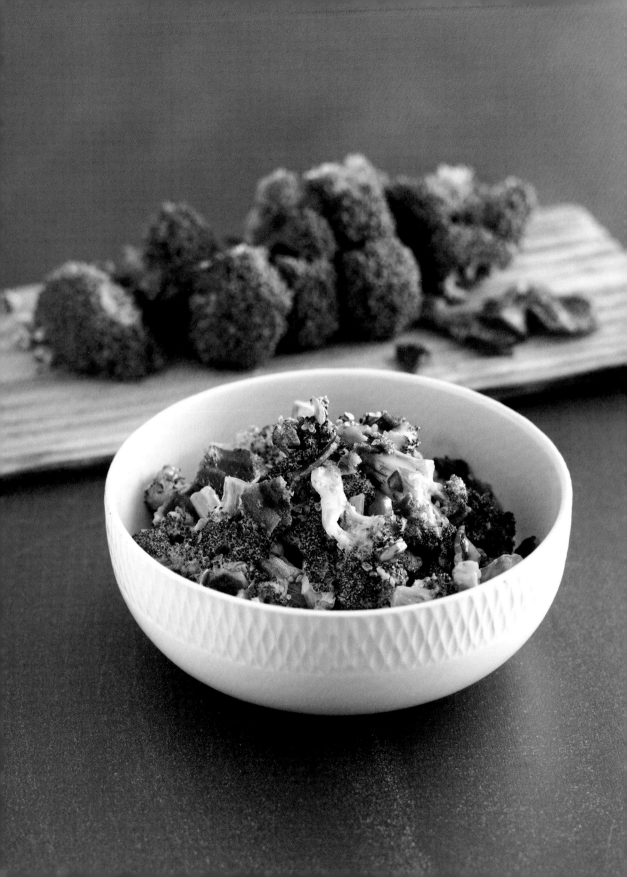

Bacon Broccoli Salad

Do you think salad means boring lettuce and a few tasteless toppings? Think again! The beauty of keto is getting to load up your salads with so many flavorful veggies that you can sometimes even skip the lettuce. This salad will refresh you if you're stuck in a salad rut.

- **Hands-on time:** 10 minutes
- **Cook time:** 10 minutes

Serves 4

6 slices bacon

4 cups fresh broccoli, chopped

¼ cup mayo

3 tablespoons Thai chili sauce

2 tablespoons pepitas

WHAT ARE PEPITAS?

Pepitas are pumpkin seeds. They're generally smaller and flatter than seeds you might find in a pie pumpkin. The seeds you find inside carving pumpkins have a shell on them, so you usually can't see the darker colored pepita inside.

1 Press the Sauté button and add bacon to Instant Pot®. Cook bacon until crisp.

2 When bacon is cooked, remove and place on paper towel until cool. Add broccoli into bacon grease and stir-fry for 3 minutes until just beginning to soften. Press the Cancel button.

3 Remove broccoli and place in large bowl to set aside. In small bowl, mix mayo and chili sauce. Add sauce mixture to large bowl. Crumble bacon over bowl and toss. Sprinkle pepitas on top to serve. Serve warm or cold.

CALORIES: 319

PROTEIN: 7.9 grams

FIBER: 0.4 grams

NET CARBOHYDRATES: 10.3 grams

FAT: 26.2 grams

SODIUM: 463 milligrams

CARBOHYDRATES: 10.7 grams

SUGAR: 5.0 grams

Classic Deviled Eggs

This classic party dish is a perfect keto snack. It's loaded with fats and protein to keep you going. Feel free to customize it with your favorite flavors such as bacon, or simply enjoy it as is.

- **Hands-on time:** 15 minutes
- **Cook time:** 8 minutes

Serves 3

6 eggs
1 cup water
¼ cup mayo
½ teaspoon salt
⅛ teaspoon pepper
½ teaspoon yellow mustard
¼ teaspoon paprika

1 Place eggs on steamer basket and add to Instant Pot®. Pour water into pot and click lid closed. Press the Egg button and adjust time for 8 minutes.

2 When timer beeps, quick-release the pressure and remove steamer basket. Place eggs in cold water and peel when cooled. Slice eggs in half lengthwise.

3 Remove yolks and set egg whites aside. Place yolks, mayo, salt, pepper, and mustard in food processor and blend until smooth. (Alternatively, press with fork until all ingredients are smooth.) Place filling into egg whites. Sprinkle with paprika and refrigerate at least 30 minutes or until chilled.

CALORIES: 268	**FAT:** 22.1 grams
PROTEIN: 12.8 grams	**SODIUM:** 650 milligrams
FIBER: 0.1 grams	**CARBOHYDRATES:** 1.0 grams
NET CARBOHYDRATES: 0.9 grams	**SUGAR:** 0.5 grams

Blackened Chicken Bites and Ranch

This is a great on-the-go snack. The spiciness from the chicken paired with the cooling ranch is a winning duo. Gone are the days of stopping to get high-carb chicken nuggets while you're out for the day, so this quick fix is a great alternative.

- **Hands-on time: 5 minutes**
- **Cook time: 15 minutes**

Serves 1

2 ounces boneless, skinless chicken breast, cubed
¼ teaspoon dried thyme
¼ teaspoon paprika
¼ teaspoon pepper
¼ teaspoon garlic powder
3 tablespoons coconut oil
½ cup ranch dressing
2 tablespoons hot sauce

1 Toss chicken pieces in seasonings. Press the Sauté button and add coconut oil to Instant Pot®. Sear chicken until dark golden brown and thoroughly cooked.

2 To make sauce, remove chicken from Instant Pot® and press the Cancel button. Pour ranch and hot sauce into Instant Pot®. Use wooden spoon to scrape any seasoning from bottom of pot. Heat on Keep Warm for 5 minutes. Pour into small bowl for serving. Serve chicken bites warm with dipping sauce.

CALORIES: 228
PROTEIN: 6.8 grams
FIBER: 0.3 grams
NET CARBOHYDRATES: 0.7 grams

FAT: 21.4 grams
SODIUM: 135 milligrams
CARBOHYDRATES: 1.0 grams
SUGAR: 0.2 grams

Boiled Peanuts

This flavorful snack is better homemade—sometimes storebought versions contain large amounts of sodium and preservatives. There's no limit to how many ways these peanuts can be customized, from something spicy (by adding pepper flakes while they boil) to something sweet (by adding sugar-free chocolate chips or a natural sweetener like erythritol). This recipe will give you the base instructions, but feel free to explore the possibilities!

- **Hands-on time:** 5 minutes
- **Cook time:** 60 minutes

Makes 4 servings; serving size 1 cup (shell on)

2 pounds raw green peanuts in shell

1 cup water

¼ cup salt

1 Add all ingredients to Instant Pot®. Peanuts will float, so place steam rack or steamer basket upside down on top of peanuts. (Place a small Instant Pot®–safe bowl on top to weigh down steamer basket and prevent floating.)

2 Press the Manual button and adjust time for 60 minutes. When timer beeps, allow a 20-minute natural release and then quick-release the remaining pressure.

CALORIES: 200

PROTEIN: 8.5 grams

FIBER: 5.5 grams

NET CARBOHYDRATES: 7.9 grams

FAT: 13.2 grams

SODIUM: 473 milligrams

CARBOHYDRATES: 13.4 grams

SUGAR: 1.6 grams

Savory Snack Mix

Part of success on a keto diet is getting creative with your snacks. You find all sorts of hacks and flavor combos you wouldn't think to normally try. Pork rinds are surprisingly versatile and with the right seasoning, they can become the crunch you might have been missing.

- **Hands-on time: 5 minutes**
- **Cook time: 2 hours**

Serves 8

2 cups whole almonds
2 cups pork rinds
½ cup pecans
4 tablespoons butter
1 teaspoon chili powder
½ teaspoon garlic powder
⅛ teaspoon cayenne

Place all ingredients into Instant Pot®, place slow cooker lid on pot, and press the Slow Cook button. Slow cook for 2 hours, stirring occasionally.

CALORIES: 321	FAT: 27.8 grams
PROTEIN: 10.4 grams	SODIUM: 75 milligrams
FIBER: 5.2 grams	CARBOHYDRATES: 8.9 grams
NET CARBOHYDRATES: 3.7 grams	SUGAR: 1.8 grams

Pickled Jalapeño and Bacon Dip

This dip is spicy, but the flavors are balanced by the cool and creamy mayo. It's a quick snack but can also be a great small meal with low-carb veggies to dip.

- **Hands-on time: 3 minutes**
- **Cook time: 3 minutes**

Serves 6; serving size ¼ cup

½ cup pickled jalapeños
½ cup mayo
1 clove garlic, finely minced
8 ounces cream cheese
½ cup cooked crumbled bacon
½ cup Chicken Broth (see recipe in Chapter 3)

Add all ingredients to Instant Pot®. Click lid closed. Adjust time for 3 minutes. Quick-release the pressure when timer beeps.

CALORIES: 354	FAT: 29.9 grams
PROTEIN: 8.2 grams	SODIUM: 614 milligrams
FIBER: 0.6 grams	CARBOHYDRATES: 8.1 grams
NET CARBOHYDRATES: 7.5 grams	SUGAR: 6.7 grams

Sweet Snack Mix

This is the perfect mix for movie night or anytime you just want something sweet. This is a great mix of salty and sweet that can help you get over that sweet tooth hurdle without getting off track. You can even sprinkle this mix on top of a low-carb yogurt.

- **Hands-on time: 5 minutes**
- **Cook time: 2 hours**

Serves 8

2 cups pork rinds

1 cup pecans

½ cup almonds

½ cup flaked unsweetened coconut

4 tablespoons butter

½ cup powdered erythritol

2 egg whites

½ teaspoon cinnamon

2 teaspoons vanilla extract

¼ cup low-carb chocolate chips

1 Break pork rinds into bite-sized pieces and place into Instant Pot®. Press the Sauté button and add pecans, almonds, coconut flakes, and butter. Cook 2–4 minutes until butter is completely melted. Press the Cancel button.

2 In medium bowl, whip erythritol, egg whites, cinnamon, and vanilla until soft peaks form. Slowly add to Instant Pot®. Gently fold mixture into ingredients already in pot. Place slow cooker lid on pot and press the Slow Cook button. Adjust time for 2 hours. Stir every 20–30 minutes.

3 When mixture is dry and crunchy, place on parchment-lined baking sheet to cool. Once cooled fully, sprinkle with chocolate chips and store in sealed container.

CALORIES: 274

PROTEIN: 6.4 grams

FIBER: 3.4 grams

NET CARBOHYDRATES: 2.6 grams

SUGAR ALCOHOLS: 12.5 grams

FAT: 23.9 grams

SODIUM: 80 milligrams

CARBOHYDRATES: 18.5 grams

SUGAR: 1.3 grams

5

Side Dishes

Have you been browsing mouthwatering, low-carb entrée recipes and asking yourself, "What would go with that?" Just because you stopped pairing your meals with traditional staples like rice and potatoes doesn't mean you have to miss out on flavorful, filling side dishes for your ketogenic dinners. Get ready to serve up vegetable dishes that you and your family will be excited to eat. Plus, your Instant Pot® will save you time by cooking these sides in minutes! This chapter includes easy sides like Garlic Butter Steamed Broccoli and Perfect Zucchini Noodles to help complete your meals with plenty of vitamins and nutrients.

Salsa Verde

This tangy and spicy salsa is perfect on its own or in your favorite taco dish. Its deep yet fresh flavor is unique and a great way to change things up from your traditional salsa. If you'd like something spicier, leave more seeds in the peppers. For a more mild taste, remove all the seeds.

- **Hands-on time:** 5 minutes
- **Cook time:** 25 minutes

Makes 2½ cups; serving size ½ cup

1 pound tomatillos
3 cloves garlic
2 whole serrano peppers
2 whole jalapeños
½ medium onion, chopped
1 teaspoon salt
¼ cup chopped cilantro
1 cup Chicken Broth (see recipe in Chapter 3)
¼ teaspoon xanthan gum
2 teaspoons avocado oil

1 Remove husks from tomatillos. Peel garlic. Slice jalapeños and serrano peppers in half lengthwise, cut off stems, and remove most seeds. Peel and chop onion. Place all into Instant Pot®.

2 Add salt, cilantro, and Chicken Broth to Instant Pot®. Click lid to close. Press the Manual button and set timer to 10 minutes. When timer goes off, natural-release the pressure for 5 minutes. Quick-release the remaining steam.

3 Pour Instant Pot® contents into food processor and pulse until desired texture. Stir in xanthan gum and allow a few minutes to thicken. Return mixture to Instant Pot® and press the Sauté button. Add avocado oil. Allow salsa to reduce for 15 minutes. Store in sealed container in fridge.

CALORIES: 58
PROTEIN: 1.5 grams
FIBER: 2.4 grams
NET CARBOHYDRATES: 5.3 grams
FAT: 6.6 grams
SODIUM: 468 milligrams
CARBOHYDRATES: 7.7 grams
SUGAR: 4.4 grams

Barbecue Sauce

In most cases a good barbecue sauce is packed full of sugar, sugar, and more sugar. This special flavor is a key part of so many popular recipes, including several in this book, so it's essential to have a good sauce recipe that's actually low-carb! With just a few simple ingredients you can easily whip up a tangy barbecue sauce in your Instant Pot® that you can jar and refrigerate. It will keep for one week in the fridge.

- **Hands-on time:** 5 minutes
- **Cook time:** 10 minutes

Makes 2 cups; serving size 2 tablespoons

1 cup reduced-sugar ketchup
½ cup tomato paste
½ cup water
3 tablespoons apple cider vinegar
2 teaspoons erythritol
½ teaspoon garlic powder
½ teaspoon liquid smoke
½ teaspoon Worcestershire sauce
⅛ teaspoon guar gum

Press the Sauté button and press the Adjust button to set heat to Less. Place all ingredients in Instant Pot®. Simmer until fragrant and begins to thicken.

CALORIES: 17	**FAT:** 0.0 grams
PROTEIN: 0.7 grams	**SODIUM:** 267 milligrams
FIBER: 0.4 grams	**CARBOHYDRATES:** 3.2 grams
NET CARBOHYDRATES: 2.3 grams	**SUGAR:** 1.0 grams
SUGAR ALCOHOLS: 0.5 grams	

MORE ON GUAR GUM

Guar gum is a stabilizer that can help thicken sauces. You can typically find it in the baking aisle near the yeast and xanthan gum. It often comes in small packets, but you can also find it in larger bags at health food stores.

Sautéed Radishes

You may have only tried radishes raw in a salad, but sautéing them brings out a whole new flavor. They're transformed from peppery and zesty when fresh, to mild with a hint of sweetness when sautéed. Savory herbs and butter make this side dish a nice break from all the green veggies you're likely to be eating.

- **Hands-on time:** 5 minutes
- **Cook time:** 15 minutes

Serves 4

1 pound radishes, quartered
  (remove leaves and ends)
2 tablespoons butter
¼ teaspoon dried thyme
¼ teaspoon minced garlic
⅛ teaspoon salt
⅛ teaspoon garlic powder
⅛ teaspoon dried rosemary

1 Press the Sauté button and then press the Adjust button to lower heat to Less.

2 Place radishes into Instant Pot® with butter and seasoning.

3 Sauté, stirring occasionally until tender, about 10–15 minutes. Add a couple of teaspoons of water if radishes begin to stick.

CALORIES: 62

FAT: 5.4 grams

PROTEIN: 0.6 grams

SODIUM: 101 milligrams

FIBER: 1.2 grams

CARBOHYDRATES: 2.6 grams

NET CARBOHYDRATES: 1.4 grams

SUGAR: 1.3 grams

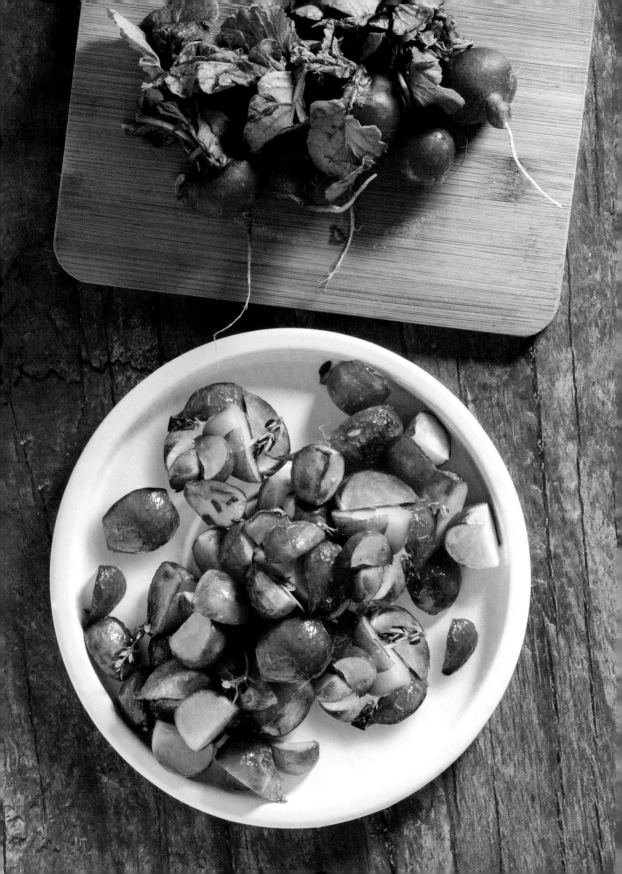

Quick Steamed Cauliflower

This simple recipe can be eaten as a side dish or become the base for a bunch of delicious dishes. From cauliflower rice to cauliflower mash to cauliflower mac and cheese, it is extremely versatile. If you're eating this as a side dish, add a bit of butter and your favorite herb mixture such as garlic and Parmesan or chili powder and crushed red pepper. You'll find that this dish can accompany a wide variety of meals and be a great way to increase your fat for the day.

- **Hands-on time: 3 minutes**
- **Cook time: 1 minute**

Serves 2

1 cup water
½ large head of cauliflower, chopped

1 Add water to Instant Pot® and place steamer basket inside pot. Put cauliflower into steamer basket.

2 Click lid closed. Press the Steam button and adjust time for 1 minute. When timer beeps, quick-release the steam. When pressure indicator drops, remove steamer basket. Feel free to season with your choice of herbs, salt, and butter (adjust the nutritional stats accordingly).

CALORIES: 52
PROTEIN: 4.0 grams
FIBER: 4.2 grams
NET CARBOHYDRATES: 6.2 grams

FAT: 0.4 grams
SODIUM: 62 milligrams
CARBOHYDRATES: 10.4 grams
SUGAR: 4.0 grams

Perfect Zucchini Noodles

Zucchini noodles, also known as "zoodles," are a popular way to replace traditional pasta. Running zucchini through a spiralizer gives you spaghetti-like strands in minutes.

- **Hands-on time:** 5 minutes
- **Cook time:** 4 minutes

Serves 2

1 tablespoon coconut oil
2 large zucchini, spiralized
½ teaspoon salt

1   Press the Sauté button and press the Adjust button to set heat to Less. Add coconut oil to Instant Pot®.

2   Sprinkle zucchini with salt. Toss in coconut oil until just beginning to soften, 3–6 minutes, depending on zoodle thickness. (Watch them carefully—overcooking will cause them to release excess water and get soggy.) Serve warm in favorite sauce.

CALORIES: 113	**FAT:** 7.0 grams
PROTEIN: 3.9 grams	**SODIUM:** 606 milligrams
FIBER: 3.2 grams	**CARBOHYDRATES:** 10.1 grams
NET CARBOHYDRATES: 6.9 grams	**SUGAR:** 8.1 grams

Basic Spaghetti Squash

Spaghetti squash is an excellent alternative to traditional pasta in a ketogenic diet. Your Instant Pot® can help you create this delicious base for a savory Italian meal with a great taste, pleasant texture, and a fraction of the carbs! Be sure to try the Spaghetti Squash Casserole in Chapter 7 too.

- **Hands-on time:** 3 minutes
- **Cook time:** 9 minutes

Serves 2

1 spaghetti squash
1 cup water

1   Carefully cut squash in half lengthwise. Scoop out seeds. Place halves on steam rack in Instant Pot®. Press the Manual button and set timer for 9 minutes.

2   When done, quick-release the pressure. Use fork to pull strands. Serve warm with favorite low-carb sauce or butter.

CALORIES: 104	**FAT:** 0.8 grams
PROTEIN: 2.6 grams	**SODIUM:** 69 milligrams
FIBER: 5.4 grams	**CARBOHYDRATES:** 25.0 grams
NET CARBOHYDRATES: 19.6 grams	**SUGAR:** 9.8 grams

Garlic Butter Steamed Broccoli

This savory broccoli is the perfect companion for any meaty entrée. Rich with vitamins, fiber, and phytonutrients, this is a side you'll always feel good about eating.

- **Hands-on time:** 3 minutes
- **Cook time:** 1 minute

Serves 2

1 cup water
2 cups broccoli, chopped
½ teaspoon salt
½ teaspoon garlic powder
2 tablespoons butter

1 Add water to Instant Pot® and place steamer basket inside pot. Add broccoli to basket.

2 Click lid closed. Press the Steam button and adjust time for 1 minute. When timer beeps, quick-release the steam. Wait until pressure indicator drops and open lid.

3 Remove basket and place broccoli in large bowl. Sprinkle with salt and garlic powder. Toss with butter until melted. Serve warm.

CALORIES: 123
PROTEIN: 2.4 grams
FIBER: 0.1 grams
NET CARBOHYDRATES: 4.2 grams
FAT: 10.9 grams
SODIUM: 601 milligrams
CARBOHYDRATES: 4.3 grams
SUGAR: 0.0 grams

Italian Zucchini

The right flavor profile is usually all you need to turn a vegetable dish from boring to delicious, and this recipe gets it right! The Italian seasoning provides just the right amount of flavor, and none of the carbs.

- **Hands-on time:** 5 minutes
- **Cook time:** 10 minutes

Serves 4

3 large zucchini, chopped
1 clove garlic, finely minced
2 tablespoons avocado oil
½ teaspoon salt
¼ teaspoon oregano
½ teaspoon basil
¼ teaspoon garlic powder
½ cup Easy Tomato Sauce
    (see recipe in Chapter 4)

Add all ingredients to Instant Pot® and press the Sauté button. Sauté 10 minutes. Serve warm.

CALORIES: 136
PROTEIN: 3.9 grams
FIBER: 3.2 grams
NET CARBOHYDRATES: 8.2 grams
FAT: 8.9 grams
SODIUM: 444 milligrams
CARBOHYDRATES: 11.4 grams
SUGAR: 8.3 grams

Bacon Brussels Sprouts

Remember being a kid and having your parents tell you to eat your Brussels sprouts while you pushed a tasteless serving of them around your plate? When you bite into this dish, you'll wish you had been served these Brussels sprouts all along! It's rich in nutrients, including heart-healthy omega-3 fatty acids, and cooked with savory bacon. Say hello to a side the whole family will be happy about!

- **Hands-on time: 5 minutes**
- **Cook time: 10 minutes**

Serves 4

½ pound bacon
1 pound Brussels sprouts
4 tablespoons butter
1 teaspoon salt
½ teaspoon pepper
½ cup water

FLAVOR BOOST

For an added burst of salty flavor, try adding a splash of soy sauce or liquid aminos. For an Italian twist, you can add a pinch of garlic and serve with Italian-seasoned chicken.

1 Press the Sauté button and press the Adjust button to lower heat to Less. Add bacon to Instant Pot® and fry for 3–5 minutes or until fat begins to render. Press the Cancel button.

2 Press the Sauté button, with heat set to Normal, and continue frying bacon until crispy. While bacon is frying, wash Brussels sprouts and remove damaged outer leaves. Cut in half or quarters.

3 When bacon is done, remove and set aside. Add Brussels sprouts to hot bacon grease and add butter. Sprinkle with salt and pepper. Sauté for 8–10 minutes until caramelized and crispy, adding a few tablespoons of water at a time as needed to deglaze pan. Serve warm.

CALORIES: 387	FAT: 32.1 grams
PROTEIN: 11.1 grams	SODIUM: 986 milligrams
FIBER: 4.4 grams	CARBOHYDRATES: 11.1 grams
NET CARBOHYDRATES: 6.7 grams	SUGAR: 3.1 grams

Creamed Spinach

This recipe adds a richness to the flavor profile of the very nutritious and fiber-rich spinach. Even better, the creaminess makes spinach more fun to eat, and even frozen spinach steams up beautifully in the Instant Pot®. Make this recipe as a side for your favorite chicken dish to round out the meal in a luscious and healthy way. Fry a couple slices of bacon and sprinkle on top for an extra crunch with your dish!

- **Hands-on time: 3 minutes**
- **Cook time: 5 minutes**

Serves 6

4 tablespoons butter

¼ cup diced onion

8 ounces cream cheese

1 (12-ounce) bag frozen spinach

½ cup Chicken Broth (see recipe in Chapter 3)

1 cup shredded whole-milk mozzarella cheese

1 Press the Sauté button and add butter. Once butter is melted, add onion to Instant Pot® and sauté for 2 minutes or until onion begins to turn translucent.

2 Break cream cheese into pieces and add to Instant Pot®. Press the Cancel button. Add frozen spinach and broth. Click lid closed. Press the Manual button and adjust time for 5 minutes. When timer beeps, quick-release the pressure and stir in shredded mozzarella. If mixture is too watery, press the Sauté button and reduce for additional 5 minutes, stirring constantly.

CALORIES: 273

PROTEIN: 8.7 grams

FIBER: 1.8 grams

NET CARBOHYDRATES: 3.2 grams

FAT: 23.9 grams

SODIUM: 298 milligrams

CARBOHYDRATES: 5.0 grams

SUGAR: 2.1 grams

Buttery Spinach

Spinach contains omega-3, which helps reduce inflammation and is an excellent source of vitamin K, vitamin C, and iron. This dish is great for using up greens that have started to wilt.

- **Hands-on time: 5 minutes**
- **Cook time: 10 minutes**

Serves 2

4 cups fresh spinach
4 tablespoons butter
½ teaspoon salt
¼ teaspoon pepper
¼ teaspoon garlic powder
⅛ teaspoon red pepper flakes

Press the Sauté button and press the Adjust button to set heat to Less. Place all ingredients in Instant Pot® and sauté until greens are soft, approximately 10 minutes.

CALORIES: 218		**FAT:** 21.6 grams	
PROTEIN: 2.1 grams		**SODIUM:** 631 milligrams	
FIBER: 1.4 grams		**CARBOHYDRATES:** 2.7 grams	
NET CARBOHYDRATES: 1.3 grams		**SUGAR:** 0.3 grams	

Buttery Cabbage

Cabbage is an often-overlooked vegetable, but did you know that it's loaded with vitamins, fiber, calcium, and potassium? It's an excellent keto option that's definitely worth eating more of! This simple, buttery cabbage shows you how to achieve the perfect tenderness while cooking a head of cabbage.

- **Hands-on time: 5 minutes**
- **Cook time: 5 minutes**

Serves 4

1 medium head white cabbage, sliced into strips
4 tablespoons butter
½ teaspoon salt
¼ teaspoon pepper
1 cup water

1 Place cabbage in 7-cup glass bowl with butter, salt, and pepper.

2 Pour water into Instant Pot® and place steam rack on bottom. Place bowl on steam rack. Click lid closed. Press the Manual button and adjust time for 5 minutes. When timer beeps, quick-release the pressure.

CALORIES: 158		**FAT:** 10.8 grams	
PROTEIN: 3.0 grams		**SODIUM:** 332 milligrams	
FIBER: 5.7 grams		**CARBOHYDRATES:** 13.3 grams	
NET CARBOHYDRATES: 7.6 grams		**SUGAR:** 7.3 grams	

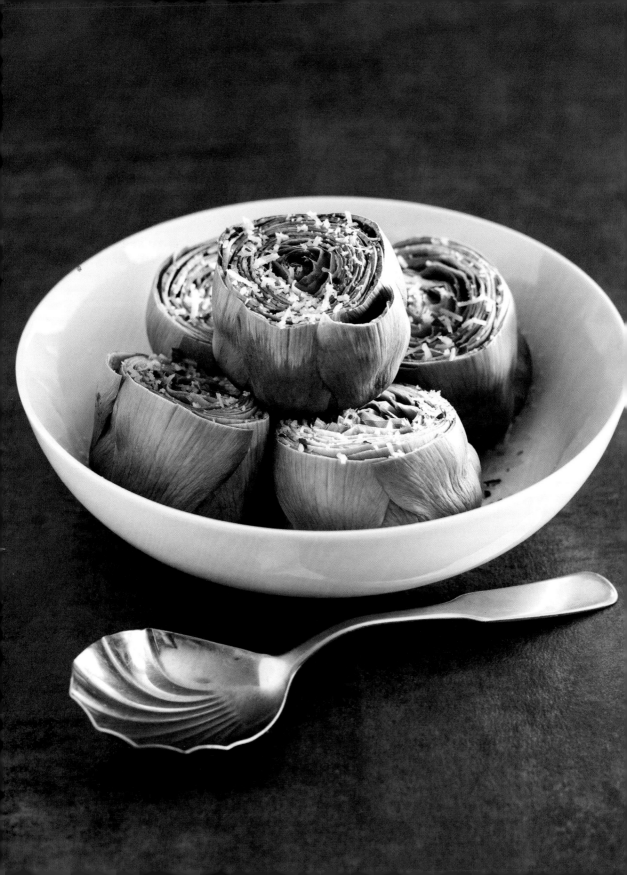

Steamed Artichoke

Artichokes are a low-carb, low-calorie vegetable, and a great source of potassium, vitamin C, and dietary fiber. With this mountain of benefits, they're hard not to love, and steaming them is an easy way to get them ready to eat with all of the nutrients intact!

- **Hands-on time:** 1 minute
- **Cook time:** 30 minutes

Serves 2

1 large artichoke
1 cup water
¼ cup grated Parmesan cheese
¼ teaspoon salt
¼ teaspoon red pepper flakes

1 Trim artichoke. Remove stem, outer leaves and top. Gently spread leaves.

2 Add water to Instant Pot® and place steam rack on bottom. Place artichoke on steam rack and sprinkle with Parmesan, salt, and red pepper flakes. Click lid closed. Press the Steam button and adjust time for 30 minutes.

3 When timer beeps, allow a 15-minute natural release and then quick-release the remaining pressure. Enjoy warm topped with additional parmesan.

CALORIES: 90
PROTEIN: 6.2 grams
FIBER: 4.4 grams
NET CARBOHYDRATES: 5.9 grams
FAT: 3.1 grams
SODIUM: 592 milligrams
CARBOHYDRATES: 10.3 grams
SUGAR: 0.8 grams

Pesto Zucchini Noodles

Pesto is a fresh-tasting, savory green sauce native to Italy. It can be found in many Italian recipes, especially pastas, but it also pairs great with low-carb alternatives like zucchini noodles. Pesto is very low-carb on its own, so keeping a jar in your fridge for easy access is a smart way to add flavor in a flash!

- **Hands-on time:** 5 minutes
- **Cook time:** 3 minutes

Serves 2

2 large zucchini, spiralized
½ teaspoon salt
¼ teaspoon pepper
2 tablespoons butter
¼ cup pesto
⅛ cup grated Parmesan

1 Sprinkle zucchini with salt and pepper. Press the Sauté button and add butter to Instant Pot®. Let butter melt then add spiralized zucchini. Sauté for 2–3 minutes only. (Overcooking them will cause them to release excess water and get soggy.)

2 Press the Cancel button and add pesto. Sprinkle with grated Parmesan. Serve warm.

CALORIES: 182
PROTEIN: 7.3 grams
FIBER: 3.8 grams
NET CARBOHYDRATES: 10.3 grams

FAT: 23.2 grams
SODIUM: 1,080 milligrams
CARBOHYDRATES: 14.1 grams
SUGAR: 9.1 grams

CHOOSING THE RIGHT SPIRALIZER

You can find many types of spiralizers, including handheld and larger ones that mount onto the countertop. Handheld ones are great if you are cooking for yourself or don't eat zoodles often. If you are making more for a family, you may want to invest in a larger one. They generally cost under $20.

Cheesy Cauliflower Rice

Swapping out traditional rice for cauliflower in this easy, cheesy dish makes it a low-carb side you can enjoy as often as you like while maintaining your keto diet. Want to feel even better about this healthy choice? One cup of cauliflower has just about 10 percent of the total carbs in the same amount of white rice! Now that's a smart swap.

- **Hands-on time: 3 minutes**
- **Cook time: 1 minute**

Serves 4

1 head fresh cauliflower, chopped into florets

1 cup water

3 tablespoons butter

1 tablespoon heavy cream

1 cup shredded sharp cheddar cheese

½ teaspoon salt

¼ teaspoon pepper

¼ teaspoon garlic powder

1 Place cauliflower in steamer basket. Pour water into Instant Pot® and lower steamer rack into pot. Click lid closed. Press the Steam button and adjust time for 1 minute. When timer beeps, quick-release the pressure.

2 Remove steamer basket and place cauliflower in food processor. Pulse until cauliflower is broken into small pearls. Place cauliflower into large bowl, and add remaining ingredients. Gently fold until fully combined.

CALORIES: 241

PROTEIN: 9.8 grams

FIBER: 3.0 grams

NET CARBOHYDRATES: 5.0 grams

FAT: 17.9 grams

SODIUM: 518 milligrams

CARBOHYDRATES: 8.0 grams

SUGAR: 3.0 grams

CHECK THE LABEL

You may have seen premade cauliflower rice and mash products available in your grocery store. Always be sure to read the nutritional label to be sure you avoid hidden carbs or fillers.

Garlic Mashed Cauliflower

We all know mashed potatoes are a classic American staple when it comes to side dishes, but you may not know that one large potato contains a whopping 64 grams of carbs. That's definitely something you'd want to avoid on a ketogenic diet! Luckily, thanks to mashed cauliflower, you won't have to miss out on the classic side.

- **Hands-on time: 3 minutes**
- **Cook time: 1 minute**

Serves 4

1 head cauliflower, chopped into florets
1 cup water
1 clove garlic, finely minced
3 tablespoons butter
2 tablespoons sour cream
½ teaspoon salt
¼ teaspoon pepper

1. Place cauliflower on steamer rack. Add water and steamer rack to Instant Pot®. Press the Steam button and adjust time to 1 minute. When timer beeps, quick-release the pressure.

2. Place cooked cauliflower into food processor and add remaining ingredients. Blend until smooth and creamy. Serve warm.

CALORIES: 125
PROTEIN: 3.1 grams
FIBER: 3.0 grams
NET CARBOHYDRATES: 4.8 grams

FAT: 9.4 grams
SODIUM: 338 milligrams
CARBOHYDRATES: 7.8 grams
SUGAR: 3.0 grams

CUSTOMIZE IT!
Feel free to add ½ cup of your favorite shredded cheese to the mix. Not a cheese person? Try a dash of hot sauce!

Cauliflower Fried Rice

If you're a fan of Asian-inspired cuisine, you've probably been missing your fried rice since cutting the carbs. Did you know that cauliflower can replace rice in this side dish too? Cauliflower Fried Rice gives you all the savory flavors of the original without the bloat or sluggishness that can come from overindulging in carbs.

- **Hands-on time:** 5 minutes
- **Cook time:** 7 minutes

Serves 4

1 head cauliflower, chopped into florets

2 tablespoons coconut oil

¼ cup diced onion

1 clove garlic, minced

⅓ cup peas

3 tablespoons soy sauce

½ teaspoon salt

¼ teaspoon pepper

1 egg

¼ cup sliced scallions

1 Place cauliflower into food processor. Pulse until rice-like; set aside. Press the Sauté button and add coconut oil to Instant Pot®.

2 Add diced onion to Instant Pot® and sauté until translucent, about 2 minutes. Add garlic and sauté 30 seconds. Add peas and cauliflower to Instant Pot®. Stir-fry for 3–5 minutes or until cauliflower becomes slightly tender.

3 Pour soy sauce over cauliflower. Sprinkle salt and pepper. Push cauliflower to sides of Instant Pot®, leaving hole in the middle. Crack egg open into middle of pot and use fork to break up egg pieces. Using rubber spatula, gently fold cooked egg pieces into rice. Press the Cancel button and sprinkle sliced scallions on top of fried rice. Serve warm.

CALORIES: 136
PROTEIN: 6.3 grams
FIBER: 4.0 grams
NET CARBOHYDRATES: 7.5 grams

FAT: 7.9 grams
SODIUM: 1,013 milligrams
CARBOHYDRATES: 11.5 grams
SUGAR: 4.2 grams

Fresh Pumpkin Purée

Pumpkin purée is great to have as a foundation for autumn desserts and soups. Sure, you can buy a can, but if you make it, then you know exactly what's in it. Plus, sometimes the canned varieties can contain unnecessary ingredients like sugar, which is no good for keto. The Instant Pot® can cook your entire pumpkin at once!

- **Hands-on time: 1 minute**
- **Cook time: 10 minutes**

Makes 2 cups; serving size ¼ cup

1 (2–3-pound) pie pumpkin
1 cup water

HIDDEN SUGAR

Canned pumpkin purée is different from canned pumpkin pie filling. Many store-bought pumpkin pie fillings contain lots of sugar, so check your label. Better yet, make your own pumpkin pie filling! Simply follow the instructions for Fresh Pumpkin Purée then add your favorite sweetener, allspice, pumpkin spice, and cinnamon.

1 First, place pumpkin into Instant Pot® to make sure it fits. There should be no pumpkin or stem touching the lid and it should fit inside without rubbing the sides. Remove pumpkin.

2 Place steam rack into Instant Pot® and pour in water. Place pumpkin on steam rack. Press the Manual button and adjust time for 15 minutes. When timer beeps, allow a natural pressure release.

3 When pressure indicator drops, open lid and carefully remove pumpkin. Cut in half and remove seeds. It should slice open very easily. Remove pumpkin flesh and set aside to make purée.

4 Place pumpkin flesh in food processor to make purée. Purée will keep for 3 days in the refrigerator.

CALORIES: 16	FAT: 0.0 grams
PROTEIN: 0.6 grams	SODIUM: 0 milligrams
FIBER: 0.3 grams	CARBOHYDRATES: 4.1 grams
NET CARBOHYDRATES: 3.8 grams	SUGAR: 1.7 grams

Simple Cheese Sauce

Whether you're making a casserole or just need to add some excitement to steamed veggies, this sauce is the perfect sidekick. Use it as a base and add your favorite spices or switch up the cheese for a different flavor. This sauce will seem a little thicker at first, but once you incorporate it into your favorite recipes it will be the creamy, gooey cheese sauce you've always loved but without all the carbs.

- **Hands-on time: 3 minutes**
- **Cook time: 5 minutes**

Makes ¾ cup; serving size 2 tablespoons

2 tablespoons butter
2 tablespoons diced onion
1 ounce cream cheese
¼ cup heavy cream
¼ cup Chicken Broth (see recipe in Chapter 3)
⅛ teaspoon salt
⅛ teaspoon pepper
1 cup shredded cheddar cheese

1 Press the Sauté button and add butter to Instant Pot®. When butter is melted, add diced onion and sauté until onion is translucent.

2 Break cream cheese into small pieces and place around Instant Pot®. Use rubber spatula to help cream cheese melt by smoothing out pieces along bottom of pot. Add heavy cream, broth, salt, and pepper. Press the Cancel button. Stir in cheddar or cheese of choice.

CALORIES: 162	FAT: 14.8 grams
PROTEIN: 5.2 grams	SODIUM: 191 milligrams
FIBER: 0.1 grams	CARBOHYDRATES: 1.1 grams
NET CARBOHYDRATES: 1.0 grams	SUGAR: 0.6 grams

Warm Cabbage and Broccoli Slaw

Sometimes simple is best. This mix can be used as a side dish or even incorporated into a stir-fry for extra nutrients. Its buttery soft cabbage contrasts wonderfully with the bit of crunch you get from the broccoli. Try adding your favorite seasoning for a flavor profile to complement your main dish, such as a dash of soy sauce and pepper flakes or garlic powder, oregano, and parsley. You can also add shredded carrots if you want.

- **Hands-on time:** 5 minutes
- **Cook time:** 10 minutes

Serves 6

2 cups broccoli slaw
½ head cabbage, thinly sliced
¼ cup chopped kale
4 tablespoons butter
1 teaspoon salt
¼ teaspoon pepper

Press the Sauté button and add all ingredients to Instant Pot®. Stir-fry for 7–10 minutes until cabbage softens. Serve warm.

CALORIES: 97		FAT: 7.2 grams	
PROTEIN: 1.9 grams		SODIUM: 412 milligrams	
FIBER: 2.7 grams		CARBOHYDRATES: 6.5 grams	
NET CARBOHYDRATES: 3.8 grams		SUGAR: 3.0 grams	

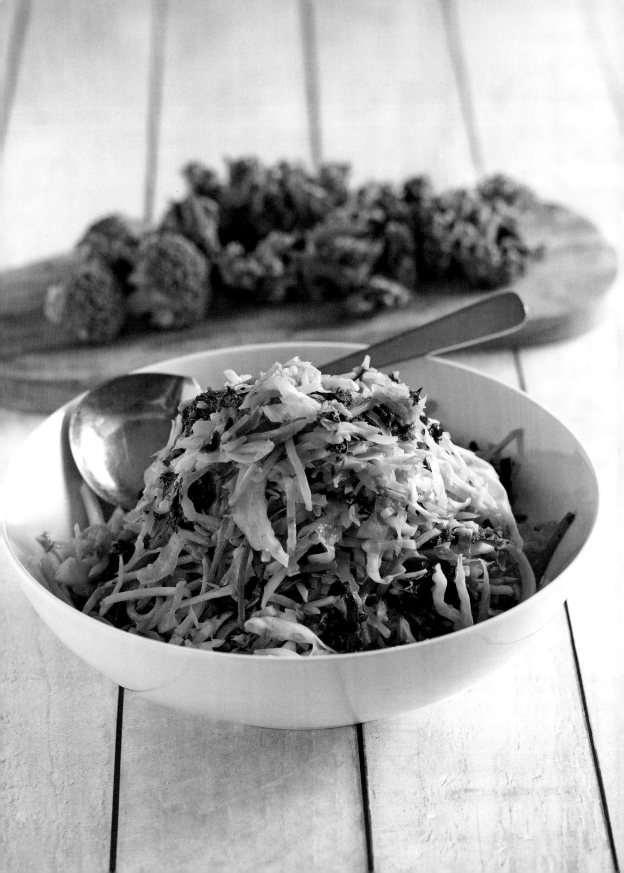

Green Bean Casserole

This creamy dish is an absolute treat for when the leaves start changing colors and it's time to put on extra layers. It's the perfect heartwarming, healthy dish to help keep your diet unhindered over the holidays! The net carbs in green beans are low so you can dive right in.

- **Hands-on time:** 5 minutes
- **Cook time:** 8 minutes

Serves 4

4 tablespoons butter

½ medium onion, diced

½ cup chopped button mushrooms

1 cup Chicken Broth (see recipe in Chapter 3)

1 teaspoon salt

¼ teaspoon pepper

1 pound green beans, edges trimmed

½ cup heavy cream

1 ounce cream cheese

¼ teaspoon xanthan gum

1 Press the Sauté button and add butter to Instant Pot®. Sauté onions and mushrooms for 3 minutes or until onions become translucent. Press the Cancel button.

2 Add broth, salt, pepper, and green beans. Click lid closed. Adjust time for 5 minutes. When timer beeps, quick-release the pressure. Stir in remaining ingredients. Serve warm.

CALORIES: 275

PROTEIN: 4.0 grams

FIBER: 3.5 grams

NET CARBOHYDRATES: 7.1 grams

FAT: 23.7 grams

SODIUM: 629 milligrams

CARBOHYDRATES: 10.6 grams

SUGAR: 5.4 grams

6

Chicken Main Dishes

There's nothing quite like sinking your teeth into a tender, juicy, perfectly seasoned piece of chicken. And, since it's one of the most popular, afford-able, and easily accessible types of meat, chicken entrées are not only essential to your family's meal rotations, but also to your ketogenic diet. Chicken is an excellent source of protein and flavor, and the Instant Pot® knows how to cook it right! Even better, you can use your Instant Pot® to cook the entire bird, so you won't have to waste a single ounce.

From the super easy Lazy Ranch Chicken made from the breasts, to the flavorful Lemon Herb Whole Chicken made from the whole bird, this chapter will inspire you to elevate your chicken dishes in practically no time at all!

Salsa Verde Chicken

Salsa Verde is a staple green sauce in many Mexican dishes that is very easy to make. When cooked with chicken, it makes for a unique flavor adventure with just the right amount of spice. Serve it inside cups of Boston lettuce for a low-carb meal.

- **Hands-on time:** 5 minutes
- **Cook time:** 12 minutes

Serves 4

1 teaspoon salt
1 teaspoon chili powder
½ teaspoon garlic powder
2 (6-ounce) boneless, skinless chicken breasts
1 tablespoon coconut oil
¼ cup Chicken Broth (see recipe in Chapter 3)
1 cup Salsa Verde (see recipe in Chapter 5)
2 tablespoons butter

CHICKEN SAFETY

Always use a meat thermometer to make sure the cooked chicken has reached an internal temperature of at least 165°F.

1 Mix seasoning together in small bowl. Sprinkle both sides of chicken with seasoning. Press the Sauté button and add coconut oil. Use tongs to place chicken into Instant Pot®.

2 Sear for 3–4 minutes, then turn and sear an additional 3–4 minutes until golden. Press the Cancel button. Add Chicken Broth and Salsa Verde. Click lid closed.

3 Press the Manual button and adjust time for 12 minutes. Allow a natural release and open lid. Remove chicken and place on cutting board. Shred chicken with fork.

4 Return chicken to warm pot, add butter, and allow to melt for additional 10 minutes.

5 Serve warm with choice of toppings, such as sour cream or shredded cheddar cheese.

CALORIES: 185	**FAT:** 13.4 grams
PROTEIN: 20.2 grams	**SODIUM:** 873 milligrams
FIBER: 1.5 grams	**CARBOHYDRATES:** 4.3 grams
NET CARBOHYDRATES: 2.8 grams	**SUGAR:** 2.3 grams

Easy Chicken for Meal Prep

If there's one meal starter staple you'll always want to keep on hand, it's this chicken. It's perfect for soups, salads, stir-fry, burrito bowls, and more. It can even be frozen for last-minute meals. Reheat it in coconut or avocado oil for a dose of heavy fat and top it with veggies for a well-rounded and easy meal.

- **Hands-on time:** 5 minutes
- **Cook time:** 10 minutes

Serves 4

1 tablespoon coconut oil
½ teaspoon garlic powder
½ teaspoon salt
½ teaspoon dried basil
½ teaspoon pepper
½ teaspoon dried oregano
2 (6-ounce) boneless,
   skinless chicken breasts
1 cup water

WHAT TO PREP?

Aim to include protein, a healthy fat, and some type of veggie in your meals. If you don't want to make distinct dishes, you can throw it all together in a salad or just build a bowl of your favorite ingredients.

1 Press the Sauté button and add coconut oil to Instant Pot®. Mix seasoning in small bowl and sprinkle evenly over chicken. Once oil is sizzling, carefully add chicken to the Instant Pot®.

2 Sear chicken for 3–4 minutes until golden on each side. Remove chicken and add water to Instant Pot®. Remove any seasoning stuck to the bottom of the pot using a rubber spatula.

3 Place steam rack inside Instant Pot® and add chicken on top of steam rack.

4 Lock lid and press the Manual button. Set timer for 10 minutes. When timer beeps, allow a natural release for 5 minutes then quick-release the remaining pressure.

5 Shred, cube, or slice chicken for salads, soups, or easy meal prep.

CALORIES: 133	**FAT:** 4.6 grams
PROTEIN: 19.3 grams	**SODIUM:** 328 milligrams
FIBER: 0.2 grams	**CARBOHYDRATES:** 0.6 grams
NET CARBOHYDRATES: 0.4 grams	**SUGAR:** 0.0 grams

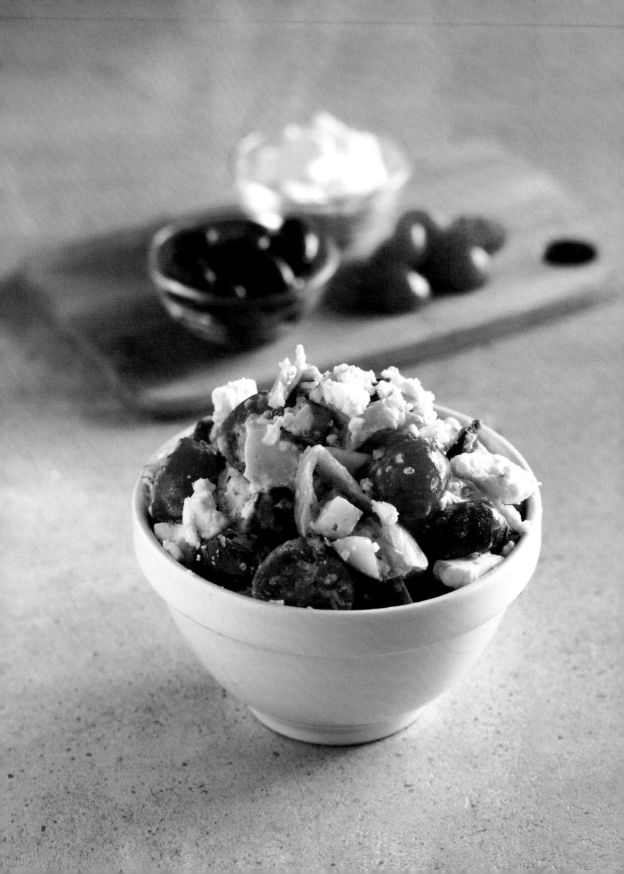

Greek Chicken Salad

An easy cold salad can be the perfect lunch on a warm afternoon. This recipe features fresh Mediterranean ingredients mixed in a zesty dressing. This is perfect for making a big batch for the week and enjoying at work for lunch or even home as a snack.

- **Hands-on time:** 2 hours
- **Cook time:** 15 minutes

Serves 4

Marinade
2 (6-ounce) boneless, skinless chicken breasts
2 garlic cloves, minced
2 tablespoons avocado oil
Juice of 1 lemon
½ teaspoon dried oregano
½ teaspoon dried thyme
¼ teaspoon salt
¼ teaspoon pepper
1 cup Chicken Broth (see recipe in Chapter 3)

Salad
¼ cup halved kalamata olives
¼ cup sliced pepperoncini
½ cup cherry tomatoes, halved
1 cup chopped cucumber
½ cup crumbled feta cheese

Dressing
½ cup mayo
¼ cup white or red wine vinegar
¼ teaspoon dried oregano
¼ teaspoon garlic powder
½ teaspoon Dijon mustard

1 Mix all marinade ingredients and chicken in resealable bag or covered container. Place in fridge to marinate for 2 hours.

2 Press the Sauté button and add chicken to Instant Pot®. Sear chicken for 3–5 minutes or until each side is browned. Add broth to pot and press the Cancel button.

3 Place lid on Instant Pot® and click to close. Press the Manual button and set timer for 10 minutes. When timer beeps, allow a natural release for 10 minutes and quick-release the remaining pressure.

4 To prepare salad, cut chicken into 1-inch bite-sized cubes. Add chicken and all salad ingredients except feta to large bowl and set aside.

5 In medium bowl, whisk together dressing ingredients and pour on top of salad, tossing to cover. Sprinkle feta on top.

CALORIES: 377
PROTEIN: 22.6 grams
FIBER: 0.5 grams
NET CARBOHYDRATES: 2.5 grams
FAT: 28.4 grams
SODIUM: 633 milligrams
CARBOHYDRATES: 3.0 grams
SUGAR: 1.9 grams

Lazy Ranch Chicken

Short on time, but looking for a meal that isn't short on flavor? This Lazy Ranch Chicken may be simple, but every bite is loaded with richness. This recipe will quickly become a weekly staple in your household if only for the amazing smells alone!

- **Hands-on time: 5 minutes**
- **Cook time: 20 minutes**

Serves 6

1 teaspoon salt

¼ teaspoon pepper

¼ teaspoon dried oregano

½ teaspoon garlic powder

3 (6-ounce) skinless chicken breasts

1 cup Chicken Broth (see recipe in Chapter 3)

1 dry ranch packet

8 ounces cream cheese

1 stick butter

PERSONALIZE IT!

There are many fun ways to personalize this dish with your favorite toppings. Try adding steamed veggies, crumbled bacon, or spice it up with a drizzle of hot sauce.

1 Mix seasoning in small bowl and sprinkle over both sides of chicken. Place chicken breasts in bottom of Instant Pot®. Place cream cheese brick and stick of butter on top of chicken breast.

2 Click lid closed. Press the Manual button and adjust time for 20 minutes. When timer beeps, allow a 10-minute natural release. Quick-release the remaining pressure.

3 Remove chicken and shred with fork. Return to Instant Pot®. Use rubber spatula to stir. Serve warm.

CALORIES: 383

PROTEIN: 21.9 grams

FIBER: 0.1 grams

NET CARBOHYDRATES: 4.5 grams

FAT: 26.9 grams

SODIUM: 926 milligrams

CARBOHYDRATES: 4.6 grams

SUGAR: 1.3 grams

Lemon Herb Whole Chicken

Busy weeknights need healthy meals too. In under 30 minutes, you can cook up a whole chicken to feed the family. The herb rub and slight hint of lemon are a great foundation for any side dish. You can use the leftover broth as a gravy or save it to make a delicious soup. Even the bones can be used later to make Bone Broth (see recipe in Chapter 3)— not a part goes to waste!

- **Hands-on time: 5 minutes**
- **Cook time: 25 minutes**

Serves 4

3 teaspoons salt
3 teaspoons garlic powder
2 teaspoons dried rosemary
2 teaspoons dried parsley
1 teaspoon pepper
1 (4–5-pound) whole chicken
2 tablespoons coconut oil
1 cup Chicken Broth (see recipe in Chapter 3)
1 lemon, zested and quartered

COOK TIME

In general, you want to cook chicken for about 6 minutes per pound in the Instant Pot®. An oven would be 20 minutes per pound, so you can really see the time savings add up!

1 In small bowl, mix salt, garlic, rosemary, parsley, and pepper. Rub herb mix over chicken. Press the Sauté button and add coconut oil to Instant Pot®. Place chicken in pot to brown for 5–7 minutes.

2 Press the Cancel button and carefully remove chicken with tongs. Add broth and scrape bottom of pot with rubber spatula or wooden spoon until no seasoning is stuck to pot. Place steam rack in pot.

3 Grate lemon zest over chicken. Place lemon quarters inside chicken. Place chicken back into Instant Pot®. Click lid closed. Press the Meat button and adjust time to 25 minutes.

4 When timer beeps, allow a 10-minute natural release and quick-release the remaining steam. Slice or shred chicken (and skin if desired); serve warm.

CALORIES: 861	**FAT:** 62.9 grams
PROTEIN: 54.5 grams	**SODIUM:** 1,963 milligrams
FIBER: 1.0 grams	**CARBOHYDRATES:** 3.1 grams
NET CARBOHYDRATES: 2.1 grams	**SUGAR:** 0.2 grams

White Chicken Casserole

You may not have noticed, but noodles don't actually have much flavor. It may seem like going pasta-less will be difficult, but you'll soon realize the most flavor is always in the *other* ingredients. This quick dish uses sliced deli chicken in place of noodles for enhanced flavor. It's still rich and packed with veggies for an incredibly filling but easy meal.

- **Hands-on time:** 15 minutes
- **Cook time:** 15 minutes

Serves 4

1 cup broccoli florets
½ cup fresh spinach
¼ cup whole-milk ricotta
1½ cups Alfredo sauce
½ teaspoon salt
¼ teaspoon pepper
1 pound thin-sliced deli
    chicken
1 cup shredded whole-milk
    mozzarella cheese
1 cup water

1. Place broccoli in large bowl. Add spinach, ricotta, Alfredo sauce, salt, and pepper to bowl and mix. Use a spoon to separate into three sections.

2. Layer chicken in bottom of 7-cup glass bowl. Place one section of the veggie mix on top in an even layer and top with a layer of mozzarella. Repeat until all veggie mix has been used and finish casserole with a layer of mozzarella.

3. Cover dish with aluminum foil. Pour water into Instant Pot® and place steam rack in bottom of pot. Place foil-covered dish on steam rack. Click lid closed. Press the Manual button and adjust time for 15 minutes.

4. When timer beeps, quick-release the pressure. If desired, broil in oven for 3–5 minutes until golden.

CALORIES: 283	**FAT:** 13.3 grams
PROTEIN: 29.3 grams	**SODIUM:** 2,321 milligrams
FIBER: 0.7 grams	**CARBOHYDRATES:** 9.8 grams
NET CARBOHYDRATES: 9.1 grams	**SUGAR:** 2.4 grams

Sweet and Sour Meatballs

This dish is often used as an appetizer, but try pairing it with sides for a weekday meal. The irresistible contrast between sweet and sour will keep everyone coming back for more.

- **Hands-on time:** 10 minutes
- **Cook time:** 10 minutes

Makes 20 meatballs; serving size 4 meatballs

1 pound ground chicken

1 egg

1 teaspoon salt

1 teaspoon pepper

1 teaspoon garlic powder

½ medium onion, diced

1 cup water

2 teaspoons erythritol

1 teaspoon rice vinegar

2 teaspoons reduced-sugar ketchup

½ teaspoon sriracha

1 Mix chicken, egg, salt, pepper, garlic powder, and onion. Form into small balls. Pour water into Instant Pot® and place steam rack on bottom. Place meatballs on steam rack.

2 Click lid closed. Press the Manual button and adjust time for 10 minutes.

3 In small bowl, mix erythritol, vinegar, ketchup, and sriracha. When timer beeps, quick-release the pressure. Toss meatballs in sauce. Serve warm.

CALORIES: 152

PROTEIN: 17.4 grams

FIBER: 0.4 grams

NET CARBOHYDRATES: 1.7 grams

SUGAR ALCOHOLS: 1.6 grams

FAT: 7.6 grams

SODIUM: 569 milligrams

CARBOHYDRATES: 3.7 grams

SUGAR: 0.8 grams

Pesto Chicken

Pesto is a wonderful alternative to white or red sauces and definitely doesn't lack in flavor. You can make your own pesto or buy store-bought versions, which are usually low in carbs. If you've never liked ricotta, you may want to try seasoning it by sprinkling herbs or salt directly on the ricotta to bring out the most flavor. The creamy element it brings to the dish is a must! Serve atop zoodles with a sprinkle of parsley.

- **Hands-on time: 5 minutes**
- **Cook time: 20 minutes**

Serves 2

2 (6-ounce) boneless, skinless chicken breasts, butterflied
½ teaspoon salt
¼ teaspoon pepper
¼ teaspoon garlic powder
¼ teaspoon dried parsley
2 tablespoons coconut oil
1 cup water
¼ cup whole-milk ricotta
¼ cup pesto
¼ cup shredded whole-milk mozzarella cheese
Chopped parsley for garnish (optional)

1 Sprinkle seasonings on chicken breasts. Press the Sauté button and add coconut oil to Instant Pot®. Sauté chicken for 3–5 minutes or until golden brown.

2 Remove chicken and place into 7-cup glass bowl. Pour water into pot and use wooden spoon or rubber spatula to make sure no seasoning is stuck to bottom of pot.

3 Place spoonful of ricotta onto chicken pieces. Pour pesto over chicken. Sprinkle mozzarella over chicken. Cover with foil. Place steam rack into Instant Pot® and carefully put bowl on top. Click lid closed. Press the Manual button and adjust time for 20 minutes. When timer beeps, allow a natural release. Serve with chopped parsley if desired.

CALORIES: 518
PROTEIN: 46.5 grams
FIBER: 0.6 grams
NET CARBOHYDRATES: 3.6 grams

FAT: 31.8 grams
SODIUM: 1,071 milligrams
CARBOHYDRATES: 4.2 grams
SUGAR: 0.2 grams

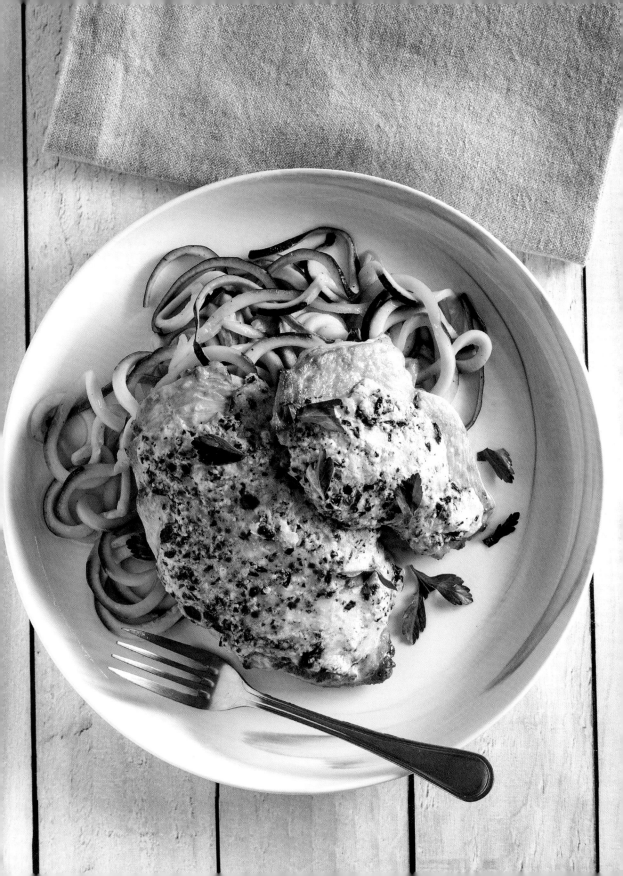

Chicken Piccata

A hint of lemon and a bite of salt from the capers make this simple dish a multi-dimensional weeknight meal. When you truly don't have the time to figure out dinner, these pantry staples will save you and help you get a great meal on the table in no time. Pair with buttery steamed broccoli or a fresh salad.

- **Hands-on time: 5 minutes**
- **Cook time: 20 minutes**

Serves 4

4 (6-ounce) boneless, skinless chicken breasts
½ teaspoon salt
¼ teaspoon pepper
½ teaspoon garlic powder
2 tablespoons coconut oil
1 cup water
4 tablespoons butter
Juice of 1 lemon
2 tablespoons capers
2 cloves garlic, minced
¼ teaspoon xanthan gum

1 Sprinkle salt, pepper, and garlic powder on chicken breast. Press the Sauté button and add coconut oil to Instant Pot®. Sear chicken until golden on each side, about 5–7 minutes. Press the Cancel button.

2 Remove chicken and set aside. Pour water into Instant Pot®; scrape bottom of pan with wooden spoon if necessary to remove any stuck-on seasoning or meat. Place steam rack in pot and add chicken.

3 Click lid closed. Press the Manual button and adjust time for 10 minutes. When timer beeps, allow a 10-minute natural release, then quick-release the remaining pressure.

4 Remove chicken and set aside. Strain broth from Instant Pot® into large bowl and return to pot. Press the Sauté button and add butter, lemon juice, capers, garlic, and xanthan gum. Stir frequently, and reduce sauce until desired thickness for at least 5 minutes. Serve over chicken.

CALORIES: 337	**FAT:** 19.5 grams
PROTEIN: 32.3 grams	**SODIUM:** 458 milligrams
FIBER: 0.5 grams	**CARBOHYDRATES:** 1.9 grams
NET CARBOHYDRATES: 1.4 grams	**SUGAR:** 0.2 grams

Garlic Parmesan Drumsticks

Drumsticks can be a pain to cook properly in the oven—they can get overcooked very easily. This Instant Pot® recipe changes all that, so you'll have tasty, fall-apart drumsticks in no time.

- **Hands-on time: 5 minutes**
- **Cook time: 15 minutes**

Serves 4

2 pounds chicken drumsticks (about 8 pieces)

1 teaspoon salt

¼ teaspoon pepper

½ teaspoon garlic powder

1 teaspoon dried parsley

½ teaspoon dried oregano

1 cup water

1 stick butter

½ cup Chicken Broth (see recipe in Chapter 3)

½ cup grated Parmesan cheese

2 ounces cream cheese, softened

¼ cup heavy cream

⅛ teaspoon pepper

1   Sprinkle seasoning evenly over drumsticks. Pour water into Instant Pot® and place steam rack into pot. Place drumsticks on steam rack and click lid closed.

2   Press the Manual button and adjust time for 15 minutes. For crispy skin, preheat oven to broil. When timer beeps, place drumsticks on foil-lined baking sheet and broil for 3–5 minutes per side or until skin begins to crisp.

3   While drumsticks are crisping, pour water out of Instant Pot®. Place pot back into heating element and press the Sauté button. Add butter to pot and let melt completely. Add broth, Parmesan, cream cheese, heavy cream, and pepper. Whisk quickly to incorporate all ingredients. Pour sauce over drumsticks and garnish with additional parsley if desired.

CALORIES: 786

PROTEIN: 53.3 grams

FIBER: 0.1 grams

NET CARBOHYDRATES: 3.4 grams

FAT: 55.4 grams

SODIUM: 1,149 milligrams

CARBOHYDRATES: 3.5 grams

SUGAR: 0.9 grams

Chicken Enchilada Bowl

This bowl is an explosion of spicy Mexican flavor. Try making a big batch at the beginning of the week to pack for lunch every day. Add a little spice by topping with jalapeños!

- **Hands-on time:** 10 minutes
- **Cook time:** 25 minutes

Serves 4

2 (6-ounce) boneless, skinless chicken breasts

½ teaspoon salt

½ teaspoon garlic powder

¼ teaspoon pepper

2 teaspoons chili powder

2 tablespoons coconut oil

¾ cup red enchilada sauce

¼ cup Chicken Broth (see recipe in Chapter 3)

¼ cup diced onion

1 (4-ounce) can green chilies

2 cups cooked cauliflower rice

1 avocado, diced

½ cup sour cream

1 cup shredded cheddar cheese

1 Sprinkle chicken with salt, garlic powder, pepper, and chili powder. Press the Sauté button and add coconut oil to Instant Pot®. Sear each side of chicken breast. Press the Cancel button.

2 Pour enchilada sauce and broth over chicken. Use wooden spoon or rubber spatula to scrape bottom of pot to make sure nothing is sticking. Add onion and chilies to pot. Click lid closed. Press the Manual button and adjust time for 25 minutes.

3 When timer beeps, quick-release the pressure and shred chicken. Serve chicken over cauliflower rice and top with diced avocado, sour cream, and cheddar.

CALORIES: 425

PROTEIN: 29.4 grams

FIBER: 4.8 grams

NET CARBOHYDRATES: 7.1 grams

FAT: 26.0 grams

SODIUM: 965 milligrams

CARBOHYDRATES: 11.9 grams

SUGAR: 5.6 grams

Loaded Buffalo Wings

Wings are always a favorite keto food. They're high in fat, moderate in protein, and zero-carb—as long as there's no hidden sugar in the sauces you add. Most sauces, such as Frank's RedHot, are acceptable. This is an exciting take on traditional buffalo wings that incorporates even more flavor to the already tasty dish.

- **Hands-on time:** 5 minutes
- **Cook time:** 12 minutes

Serves 4

2 pounds chicken wings
1 teaspoon seasoned salt
½ teaspoon garlic powder
¼ teaspoon pepper
¾ cup Chicken Broth (see recipe in Chapter 3)
¼ cup buffalo sauce
⅓ cup blue cheese crumbles
2 stalks green onion, sliced
¼ cup cooked bacon crumbles

1 Pat wings dry and sprinkle with salt, garlic, and pepper. Pour broth and buffalo sauce into Instant Pot® and place wings in bottom. Click lid closed. Press the Manual button and adjust time for 12 minutes.

2 When timer beeps, quick-release the pressure. Gently stir to coat wings with sauce.

3 For crispier wings: place on foil-lined baking sheet and broil for 3–5 minutes until skin is crispy.

4 Brush with leftover sauce and top with blue cheese, green onions, and bacon.

CALORIES: 532
PROTEIN: 46.5 grams
FIBER: 0.2 grams
NET CARBOHYDRATES: 0.9 grams

FAT: 37.0 grams
SODIUM: 1,555 milligrams
CARBOHYDRATES: 1.1 grams
SUGAR: 0.2 grams

Barbecue Wings

Some say the quality of wings can be determined by how messy your face is after you're done. These wings are dripping with zesty flavor, so you'll want a napkin close by!

- **Hands-on time:** 5 minutes
- **Cook time:** 12 minutes

Serves 4

1 pound chicken wings
1 teaspoon salt
½ teaspoon pepper
¼ teaspoon garlic powder
1 cup sugar-free barbecue sauce, divided
1 cup water

1 In bowl, toss wings in salt, pepper, garlic powder, and half of barbecue sauce. Pour water into Instant Pot®. Place steam rack on bottom of pot.

2 Place wings on steam rack and click lid closed. Press the Manual button and adjust time for 12 minutes. When timer beeps, quick-release the steam. Toss in remaining sauce.

3 For crispier wings, place on foil-lined baking sheet and broil for 5–7 minutes.

CALORIES: 237	FAT: 14.9 grams
PROTEIN: 19.9 grams	SODIUM: 1,056 milligrams
FIBER: 0.1 grams	CARBOHYDRATES: 4.3 grams
NET CARBOHYDRATES: 4.2 grams	SUGAR: 0.0 grams

Jamaican Curry Chicken

Fill your home with a Caribbean aroma as you prepare this quick and juicy Jamaican Curry Chicken. Round out the meal by serving with cauliflower rice, and don't forget to pour some of the leftover curry sauce from the pot on top!

- **Hands-on time:** 5 minutes
- **Cook time:** 20 minutes

Serves 4

1½ pounds chicken drumsticks
1 teaspoon salt
1 tablespoon Jamaican curry powder
½ medium onion, diced
½ teaspoon dried thyme
1 cup Chicken Broth (see recipe in Chapter 3)

1 Sprinkle salt and curry powder over drumsticks. Place rest of ingredients into Instant Pot®. Press the Manual button and adjust time for 20 minutes. Click lid closed.

2 When timer beeps, quick-release the pressure. Serve warm.

CALORIES: 284	FAT: 14.11 grams
PROTEIN: 31.3 grams	SODIUM: 763 milligrams
FIBER: 0.3 grams	CARBOHYDRATES: 1.7 grams
NET CARBOHYDRATES: 1.4 grams	SUGAR: 0.6 grams

Garlic Parmesan Wings

Garlic Parmesan is a milder flavor profile for wings, but don't rule it out of your rotation! This buttery, cheesy blend is a low-carb favorite at any restaurant offering wings, and your Instant Pot® version will quickly become a top rival for those chains thanks to the succulent flavor and minimal cook time.

- **Hands-on time:** 5 minutes
- **Cook time:** 12 minutes

Serves 4

2 pounds chicken wings
1 teaspoon seasoned salt
½ teaspoon pepper
½ teaspoon garlic powder
1 cup water
3 tablespoons butter
1 teaspoon lemon pepper
¼ cup grated Parmesan cheese

1 Pat wings dry and sprinkle with seasoning. Pour water into Instant Pot® and place steam rack on bottom. Place wings on steam rack and click lid closed. Press the Manual button and adjust time for 10 minutes.

2 When timer beeps, quick-release the pressure.

3 For crispy wings: place on foil-lined baking sheet and broil for 3–5 minutes.

4 Pour water out of Instant Pot®. Add butter to pot and press the Sauté button. Add lemon pepper to melted butter. Press the Cancel button. Return wings to pot and toss with tongs to completely cover with lemon pepper butter mixture. Sprinkle with Parmesan. Serve warm.

CALORIES: 536
PROTEIN: 41.7 grams
FIBER: 0.1 grams
NET CARBOHYDRATES: 1.1 grams

FAT: 39.3 grams
SODIUM: 915 milligrams
CARBOHYDRATES: 1.2 grams
SUGAR: 0.0 grams

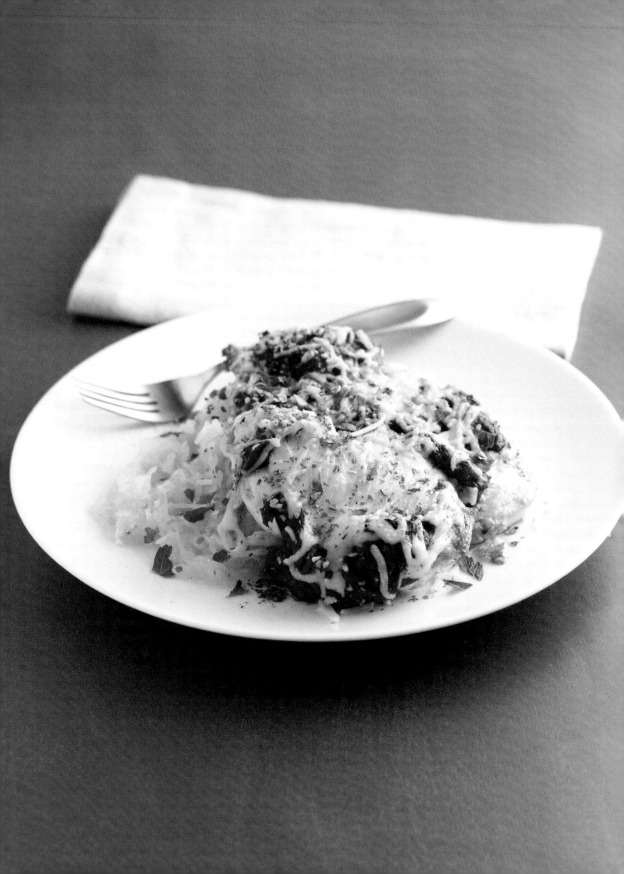

Quick Chicken Parmesan

Chicken Parmesan is a popular Italian dish that is usually made with breaded chicken covered in tomato sauce and cheese, served over spaghetti. This recipe not only cuts the carbs from the breading, but also the unnecessary sugar that is used in most tomato sauces. For a more complete dish, you can serve it over zucchini noodles or spaghetti squash.

- **Hands-on time: 5 minutes**
- **Cook time: 15 minutes**

Serves 2

2 tablespoons coconut oil
½ teaspoon salt
¼ teaspoon pepper
¼ teaspoon dried basil
½ teaspoon garlic powder
¼ teaspoon dried parsley
2 (6-ounce) boneless, skinless chicken breasts, butterflied
½ cup water
1 cup Easy Tomato Sauce (see recipe in Chapter 4)
¼ cup grated Parmesan cheese
¼ cup shredded whole-milk mozzarella cheese

1 Press the Sauté button and add coconut oil to Instant Pot®. Sprinkle seasoning evenly over chicken breasts and sear each side for 4 minutes or until golden brown. Press the Cancel button.

2 Add water and tomato sauce to Instant Pot®. Using rubber spatula or wooden spoon, scrape bottom of pot to make sure no seasoning or chicken has stuck to bottom. Click lid closed. Press the Manual button and adjust time for 15 minutes. When timer beeps, sprinkle Parmesan and mozzarella into pot and place lid on top while Instant Pot® is in warming mode for 5 minutes or until cheese has melted. Top with additional dried parsley if desired.

CALORIES: 548
PROTEIN: 48.9 grams
FIBER: 3.2 grams
NET CARBOHYDRATES: 14.1 grams
FAT: 28.7 grams
SODIUM: 1,511 milligrams
CARBOHYDRATES: 17.3 grams
SUGAR: 9.0 grams

BLT Chicken Salad

Since you won't be eating much bread on your keto diet, it's time to find a new way to satisfy your BLT cravings. This creamy salad will give you all the flavor of the classic BLT but without the carbs. The mayo adds a bit of tang and dose of fat that make this a keto-approved meal.

- **Hands-on time:** 15 minutes
- **Cook time:** 15 minutes

Serves 4

4 slices bacon
2 (6-ounce) chicken breasts
1 teaspoon salt
½ teaspoon garlic powder
¼ teaspoon pepper
¼ teaspoon dried thyme
¼ teaspoon dried parsley
1 cup water
⅓ cup mayo
1 ounce chopped pecans
½ avocado, diced
½ cup diced roma tomatoes
1 tablespoon lemon juice
2 cups chopped romaine
    lettuce

1   Press the Sauté button and press the Adjust button to set heat to Less. Add bacon to Instant Pot® and allow the fat to render for 3–5 minutes. Press the Cancel button.

2   Press the Sauté button and press the Adjust button to set heat to Normal. Finish crisping bacon; remove and set aside. Press the Cancel button. Sprinkle seasoning over chicken.

3   Pour water into Instant Pot®; use a wooden spoon to ensure nothing is stuck to the bottom. Place steam rack in pot and place chicken on top. Click lid closed. Press the Manual button and adjust time for 10 minutes.

4   While chicken is cooking, prepare sauce. In large bowl mix mayo, pecans, avocado, roma tomatoes, and lemon juice. When timer beeps, quick-release the pressure.

5   Remove chicken and let cool for 10 minutes. Then cut into cubes and add to bowl. Mix until chicken is fully coated. Mix in lettuce right before eating.

CALORIES: 430
PROTEIN: 24.4 grams
FIBER: 2.7 grams
NET CARBOHYDRATES: 2.5 grams

FAT: 32.5 grams
SODIUM: 925 milligrams
CARBOHYDRATES: 5.2 grams
SUGAR: 1.7 grams

Bacon Chicken Alfredo

Chicken, bacon, and ranch are such an awesome trifecta. There's guaranteed to be deliciousness in every bite as you dive into this creamy sauce-and-protein miracle. What a perfect way to dress your zucchini noodles!

- **Hands-on time:** 10 minutes
- **Cook time:** 20 minutes

Serves 4

2 (6-ounce) boneless, skinless chicken breasts, butterflied
¼ teaspoon salt
⅛ teaspoon pepper
½ teaspoon garlic powder
¼ teaspoon dried thyme
¼ teaspoon dried parsley
2 tablespoons coconut oil
1 cup water
1 stick butter
¼ cup heavy cream
2 cloves garlic, finely minced
½ cup grated Parmesan cheese
¼ cup cooked crumbled bacon

1 Sprinkle seasoning on chicken breasts. Press the Sauté button and add coconut oil to Instant Pot®. Sear chicken 3–5 minutes until golden brown on both sides. Press the Cancel button.

2 Remove chicken carefully using tongs, and set aside. Pour water into Instant Pot® and place steam rack in bottom.

3 Place chicken on steam rack and click lid closed. Press the Manual button and adjust time for 20 minutes. When timer beeps, quick-release the pressure. Remove chicken and set aside on clean dish.

4 Pour water out of Instant Pot®, reserving ½ cup; set aside. Press the Sauté button and add butter to pot. When butter is melted add heavy cream, garlic, Parmesan, and reserved water. Reduce for 3–4 minutes until it begins to thicken, stirring frequently. Press the Cancel button and add in cooked bacon. Pour over chicken to serve.

CALORIES: 523
PROTEIN: 27.3 grams
FIBER: 0.1 grams
NET CARBOHYDRATES: 3.0 grams
FAT: 41.2 grams
SODIUM: 611 milligrams
CARBOHYDRATES: 3.1 grams
SUGAR: 0.5 grams

Basic Taco Shredded Chicken with Fried Cheese Shells

Shredded meat is a freezer essential for making meal prep as easy as can be. In under 20 minutes, you can make a large batch of this meat and use it for the week or separate into bags for the freezer. And don't think you're restricted to just a taco bowl on the keto diet. Fried cheese shells are so delicious you'll wonder how you ever settled for traditional tortillas!

- **Hands-on time:** 5 minutes
- **Cook time:** 20 minutes

Serves 6

Chicken

1 cup Chicken Broth (see recipe in Chapter 3)
4 (6-ounce) boneless, skinless chicken breasts
1 teaspoon salt
¼ teaspoon pepper
1 tablespoon chili powder
2 teaspoons cumin
2 teaspoons garlic powder

Fried Cheese Shells

1½ cups shredded whole-milk mozzarella cheese

1 Place all chicken ingredients into Instant Pot®. Click lid closed. Press the Manual button and adjust time for 20 minutes. When timer beeps, quick-release the pressure. Shred chicken and serve in bowls or in cheese shells.

2 To make cheese shells, preheat nonstick skillet over medium on stovetop. Sprinkle ¼ cup of cheese in pan and let fry until golden. Flip and turn off heat. Allow cheese to get brown. Fill with chicken and fold. It will harden as it cools. Repeat with remaining cheese and filling. Serve warm.

CALORIES: 232	**FAT:** 8.1 grams
PROTEIN: 32.5 grams	**SODIUM:** 654 milligrams
FIBER: 0.7 grams	**CARBOHYDRATES:** 2.5 grams
NET CARBOHYDRATES: 1.8 grams	**SUGAR:** 0.5 grams

Chicken Bacon Ranch Casserole

Regular ranch dressing is actually preferred over low-fat dressings because it has less sugar and higher fat content. This flavor trifecta is a great go-to meal because it's mild, easy, and even non-low-carbers will be impressed that you can eat something so delicious.

- **Hands-on time:** 5 minutes
- **Cook time:** 20 minutes

Serves 4

4 slices bacon

4 (6-ounce) boneless, skinless chicken breasts

½ teaspoon salt

¼ teaspoon pepper

1 tablespoon coconut oil

½ cup ranch dressing

½ cup Chicken Broth (see recipe in Chapter 3)

2 ounces cream cheese

½ cup shredded cheddar cheese

1 Press the Sauté button and cook bacon until crispy; remove, and place on paper towel. While bacon is cooking, cut chicken into 1-inch bite-sized cubes, sprinkle with salt and pepper, and set aside.

2 When bacon is finished cooking, add coconut oil and chicken breasts to Instant Pot®. Sauté chicken in coconut oil and bacon grease until golden brown. Press the Cancel button.

3 Add ranch and broth. Click lid closed; press the Manual button and set time for 20 minutes. When timer beeps, quick-release the pressure and stir in cream cheese and cheddar. Crumble cooked bacon and sprinkle on top. Serve warm.

CALORIES: 466		FAT: 25.7 grams	
PROTEIN: 46.3 grams		SODIUM: 712 milligrams	
FIBER: 0.1 grams		CARBOHYDRATES: 1.4 grams	
NET CARBOHYDRATES: 1.3 grams		SUGAR: 0.9 grams	

Spinach and Feta Stuffed Chicken

Stuffed chicken sounds fancy, but it's really an easy weeknight dinner. The spinach adds powerful nutrients to this meal while balancing out the creamy feta.

- **Hands-on time:** 10 minutes
- **Cook time:** 20 minutes

Serves 4

4 (6-ounce) boneless, skinless chicken breasts, butterflied
½ cup frozen spinach
⅓ cup crumbled feta cheese
1¼ teaspoons salt, divided
¼ teaspoon pepper
¼ teaspoon garlic powder
¼ teaspoon dried oregano
¼ teaspoon dried parsley
2 tablespoons coconut oil
1 cup water

1 Pound chicken breasts to ¼-inch thickness. In medium bowl, mix frozen spinach and feta and add ¼ teaspoon salt. Evenly divide mixture and spoon onto chicken breasts.

2 Close chicken breasts and secure with toothpicks or butcher's string. Sprinkle remaining seasonings onto chicken. Press the Sauté button and add coconut oil to Instant Pot®. Sear each chicken breast until golden brown (this may take two batches). Press the Cancel button.

3 Remove chicken and set aside briefly. Pour water into Instant Pot® and scrape bottom to remove any chicken or seasoning that is stuck on. Place steam rack into pot.

4 Place chicken on steam rack and click lid closed. Adjust time for 15 minutes. When timer beeps, allow a 15-minute natural release, then quick-release the remaining pressure. Serve warm with favorite white sauce if desired.

CALORIES: 301
PROTEIN: 40.8 grams
FIBER: 0.7 grams
NET CARBOHYDRATES: 0.9 grams
FAT: 11.8 grams
SODIUM: 931 milligrams
CARBOHYDRATES: 1.6 grams
SUGAR: 0.7 grams

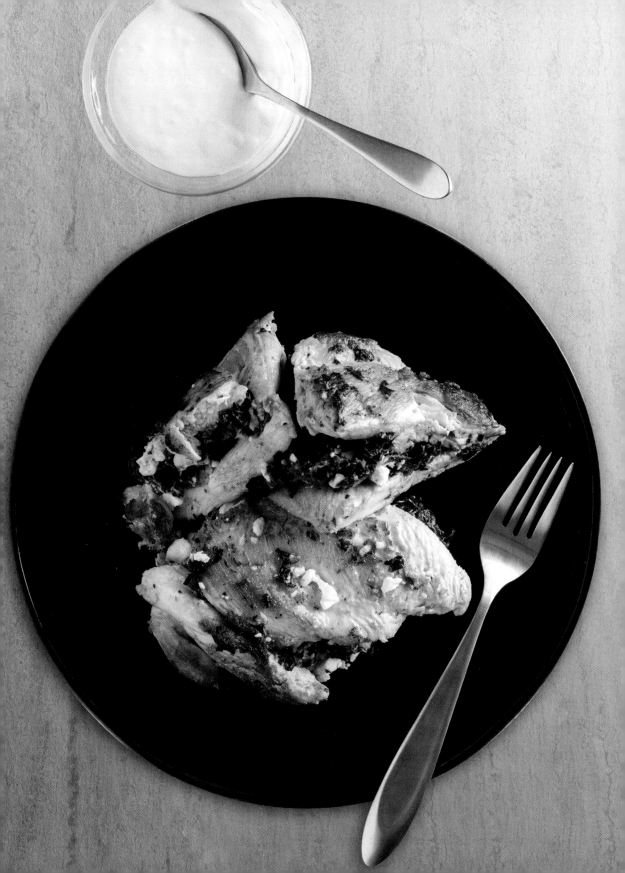

Italian Chicken Thighs

Chicken thighs are fabulous for keto cooking. They're generally the most inexpensive part of the chicken and are full of the fat that you want to help keep you full. Treat yourself to some old-fashioned thighs coated in Italian seasoning!

- **Hands-on time:** 10 minutes
- **Cook time:** 15 minutes

Serves 4

4 bone-in chicken thighs
2 cloves garlic, minced
1 teaspoon salt
¼ teaspoon pepper
¼ teaspoon dried basil
¼ teaspoon dried parsley
½ teaspoon dried oregano
1 cup water

1 Place chicken thighs in large bowl. Sprinkle with remaining ingredients except water and toss to evenly coat.

2 Pour water into Instant Pot® and place steam rack in bottom. Place chicken thighs on steam rack and click lid closed.

3 Press the Manual button and adjust time for 15 minutes. When timer beeps, quick-release the pressure. For crispy skin: broil chicken in oven for 3–5 minutes or until golden.

CALORIES: 429
PROTEIN: 32.0 grams
FIBER: 0.2 grams
NET CARBOHYDRATES: 1.0 grams

FAT: 28.8 grams
SODIUM: 737 milligrams
CARBOHYDRATES: 1.2 grams
SUGAR: 0.0 grams

Whole Barbecue Shredded Chicken

Cooking a whole chicken often means a long oven cook time, and a lot of babysitting to baste so it stays moist. Not anymore, with the Instant Pot®! Just put the ingredients in and relax. There are lots of great low-carb and sugar-free barbecue sauces at the store, so be sure to check in the health food section to find one you like.

- **Hands-on time: 5 minutes**
- **Cook time: 25 minutes**

Serves 4

1 (5-pound) whole chicken
3 teaspoons salt
1 teaspoon pepper
1 teaspoon garlic powder
1 teaspoon dried parsley
½ medium onion, cut into 3–4 large pieces
1 cup water
½ cup Barbecue Sauce (see recipe in Chapter 5), divided

1 Sprinkle chicken with salt, pepper, garlic, and parsley. Place onion pieces inside chicken cavity. Pour water into Instant Pot® and place steam rack in bottom.

2 Carefully place seasoned chicken on steam rack. Brush with half of barbecue sauce. Click lid closed.

3 Press the Manual button and adjust time for 25 minutes. When timer beeps, using a clean brush, add remaining sauce to chicken. For crispy skin or thicker sauce: broil in oven for 5 minutes or until slightly brown.

CALORIES: 1055
PROTEIN: 70.9 grams
FIBER: 1.1 grams
NET CARBOHYDRATES: 5.6 grams

FAT: 73.0 grams
SODIUM: 2,294 milligrams
CARBOHYDRATES: 6.7 grams
SUGAR: 2.2 grams

Pizza-Stuffed Chicken

Everyone is looking to spice up their chicken preparation a little bit...especially to avoid the "Chicken, again??" collective groan. There are so many ways to eliminate carbs while still maintaining traditional flavors, and this Pizza-Stuffed Chicken is a great example. Get ready for a fun chicken dinner your kids will ask for.

- **Hands-on time:** 10 minutes
- **Cook time:** 15 minutes

Serves 4

4 (6-ounce) boneless, skinless chicken breasts, butterflied

1 teaspoon salt

¼ teaspoon pepper

½ cup Easy Tomato Sauce (see recipe in Chapter 4)

16 slices pepperoni

1 cup shredded whole-milk mozzarella cheese

2 tablespoons coconut oil

1 Pound chicken breasts out until even and about ¼-inch thick. Sprinkle both sides with salt and pepper.

2 Place 2 tablespoons of sauce on each piece of chicken. Then place 4 slices of pepperoni and a quarter cup of mozzarella on each. Close each piece of chicken and secure closed with toothpicks.

3 Press the Sauté button and add coconut oil to Instant Pot®. Sear each side until golden brown. Remove chicken carefully with tongs. Pour water into Instant Pot® and add steam rack.

4 Place chicken pieces in 7-cup glass bowl. Cover with foil. Place dish on steam rack and click lid closed. Press the Manual button and adjust time for 15 minutes. When timer beeps, quick-release the pressure.

CALORIES: 428

PROTEIN: 47.3 grams

FIBER: 0.8 grams

NET CARBOHYDRATES: 3.5 grams

FAT: 20.7 grams

SODIUM: 527 milligrams

CARBOHYDRATES: 4.3 grams

SUGAR: 2.5 grams

Beef and Pork Main Dishes

Beef and pork are two of the most versatile types of meat and you can prepare them perfectly in your Instant Pot®. This chapter showcases recipes that will satisfy your family and help you hit your protein macronutrient goals. As you know, in a state of ketosis, rather than store fat in your stubborn problem areas, your body converts fat to energy that will fuel you all day long. So, embrace the fat and soak up the flavor. Get ready to dive into tons of incredible dishes, from Spicy Brisket to Chipotle Pork Chops.

Spicy Brisket

Brisket is one of those gifts that keeps on giving. The first night, dinner is amazing...and it somehow seems to taste even better the next day. The leftovers can be shredded and used for everything from pizza, to omelets, to cauliflower rice bowls. This savory herb-covered brisket is very easy to prepare. In a third of the time it takes to cook a brisket in the oven, you'll have fall-apart tender meat and a fragrant spicy broth perfect for dipping.

- **Hands-on time: 5 minutes**
- **Cook time: 110 minutes**

Serves 6

3 teaspoons salt
2 teaspoons pepper
1 teaspoon garlic powder
1 teaspoon dried thyme
½ teaspoon dried rosemary
1 (4–5-pound) beef brisket
1 tablespoon avocado oil
1 cup Beef Broth (see recipe in Chapter 3)
½ cup pickled jalapeño juice
½ cup pickled jalapeños
½ medium onion, chopped

TIP!
If your brisket is too large to fit into your Instant Pot® to brown, cut it into quarters and sear sections individually, then add all sections back to Instant Pot® for the rest of the cooking process.

1 In a small bowl combine salt, pepper, garlic powder, thyme, and rosemary. Sprinkle over brisket; set aside.

2 Press the Sauté button and add avocado oil to Instant Pot®. Sear each side of brisket for 5 minutes.

3 Add Beef Broth, jalapeño juice, jalapeños, and onions to Instant Pot®. Press the Cancel button and click to close lid.

4 Press the Manual button and adjust time to 100 minutes. When timer beeps, allow pot to naturally release, about 30–40 minutes. Don't do a quick release; it will result in tougher meat.

5 Remove brisket, slice, and pour all the strained broth over meat for additional flavor.

CALORIES: 1,001
PROTEIN: 62.0 grams
FIBER: 1.1 grams
NET CARBOHYDRATES: 8.2 grams

FAT: 68.3 grams
SODIUM: 1,746 milligrams
CARBOHYDRATES: 9.3 grams
SUGAR: 5.8 grams

Lime Pulled Pork

This pulled pork is a little smoky with a hint of spice. The tart lime and fresh cilantro brighten up the flavors. This pork would be perfect alone or added to a cauliflower rice bowl with avocado and sour cream. It freezes beautifully, making meal prep a breeze, so make sure you stock up on pork butt next time you see a good sale!

- **Hands-on time:** 5 minutes
- **Cook time:** 30 minutes

Serves 4

1 tablespoon chili adobo sauce

1 tablespoon chili powder

2 teaspoons salt

1 teaspoon garlic powder

1 teaspoon cumin

½ teaspoon pepper

1 (2½–3 pound) cubed pork butt

1 tablespoon coconut oil

2 cups Beef Broth (see recipe in Chapter 3)

1 lime, cut into wedges

¼ cup chopped cilantro

1. In a small bowl, mix adobo sauce, chili powder, salt, garlic powder, cumin, and pepper.

2. Press the Sauté button on Instant Pot® and add coconut oil to pot. Rub spice mixture onto cubed pork butt. Place pork into pot and sear for 3–5 minutes per side. Add broth.

3. Press the Cancel button. Lock Lid. Press the Manual button and adjust time to 30 minutes.

4. When timer beeps, let pressure naturally release until the float valve drops, and unlock lid.

5. Shred pork with fork. Pork should easily fall apart. For extra-crispy pork, place single layer in skillet on stove over medium heat. Cook for 10–15 minutes or until water has cooked out and pork becomes brown and crisp. Serve warm with fresh lime wedges and cilantro garnish.

CALORIES: 570

PROTEIN: 55.0 grams

FIBER: 1.1 grams

NET CARBOHYDRATES: 2.1 grams

FAT: 35.9 grams

SODIUM: 1,725 milligrams

CARBOHYDRATES: 3.2 grams

SUGAR: 0.4 grams

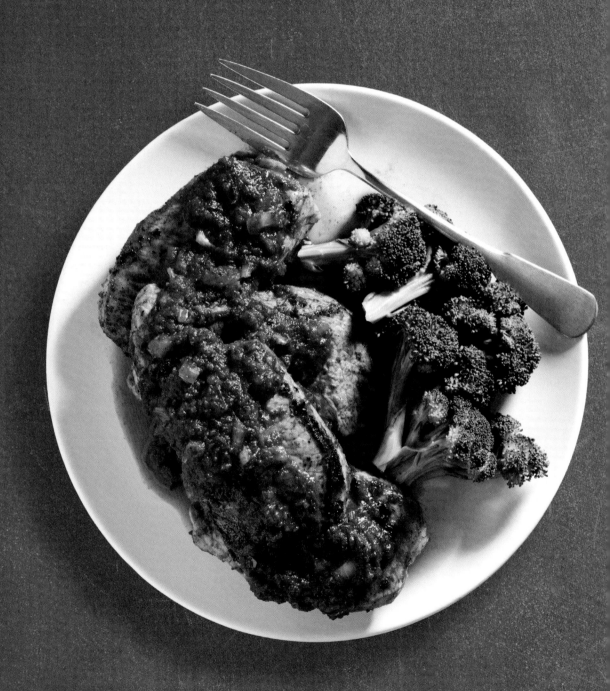

Chipotle Pork Chops

Pork chops are a great alternative to chicken when you need to mix things up. They have a deep flavor and pair well with many nutrient-rich veggies. These Chipotle Pork Chops are spiced with multiple layers of flavor that make for a filling and delectable dish. Try it alongside simple steamed broccoli.

- **Hands-on time: 7 minutes**
- **Cook time: 15 minutes**

Serves 4

2 tablespoons coconut oil
3 chipotle chilies
2 tablespoons adobo sauce
2 teaspoons cumin
1 teaspoon dried thyme
1 teaspoon salt
4 (5-ounce) boneless pork chops
½ medium onion, chopped
2 bay leaves
1 cup Chicken Broth (see recipe in Chapter 3)
½ (7-ounce) can fire-roasted diced tomatoes
⅓ cup chopped cilantro

1 Press the Sauté button and add coconut oil to Instant Pot®. While it heats, add chilies, adobo sauce, cumin, thyme, and salt to food processor. Pulse to make paste. Rub paste into pork chops. Place in Instant Pot® and sear each side 5 minutes or until browned.

2 Press the Cancel button and add onion, bay leaves, broth, tomatoes, and cilantro to Instant Pot®. Click lid closed. Press the Manual button and adjust time for 15 minutes. When timer beeps, allow a 10-minute natural release, then quick-release the remaining pressure. Serve warm with additional cilantro as garnish if desired.

CALORIES: 375	FAT: 24.2 grams
PROTEIN: 31.3 grams	SODIUM: 786 milligrams
FIBER: 1.5 grams	CARBOHYDRATES: 4.9 grams
NET CARBOHYDRATES: 3.4 grams	SUGAR: 2.0 grams

Buttery Pot Roast

Pot roast is a cold-weather staple. A hearty meal of this savory roast with a side of cauliflower mash is perfect for those cold nights. This roast is simple, flavorful, and full of fat! It's an easy go-to recipe that will have your family looking forward to dinner. With minimal prep, you can get back to the more important things like snuggling under the blanket and making memories together!

- **Hands-on time:** 5 minutes
- **Cook time:** 90 minutes

Serves 4

4 teaspoons onion powder
2 teaspoons dried parsley
1 teaspoon salt
1 teaspoon garlic powder
½ teaspoon dried oregano
½ teaspoon pepper
1 (2-pound) chuck roast
1 tablespoon coconut oil
1 cup Beef Broth (see recipe in Chapter 3)
½ packet dry ranch seasoning
1 stick butter
10 pepperoncini

1 Press the Sauté button and allow to heat. In small bowl, mix onion powder, parsley, salt, garlic powder, oregano, and pepper. Rub seasoning onto roast. Add coconut oil to Instant Pot®. Place roast in pot and sear for 5 minutes each side; remove roast and set aside.

2 Press the Cancel button. Add broth to Instant Pot®. Using rubber spatula or wooden spoon, scrape bottom to loosen any stuck-on seasoning or meat.

3 Place roast back into Instant Pot® and sprinkle dry ranch powder on top. Place stick of butter on roast and add pepperoncini. Click lid closed. Press the Manual button and adjust time for 90 minutes.

4 When timer beeps, allow a natural release to retain meat tenderness. When pressure indicator drops, remove lid and remove cooked roast. Slice or shred and top with broth from pot.

CALORIES: 561	FAT: 32.9 grams
PROTEIN: 51.2 grams	SODIUM: 1,351 milligrams
FIBER: 0.7 grams	CARBOHYDRATES: 5.8 grams
NET CARBOHYDRATES: 5.1 grams	SUGAR: 0.3 grams

Creamy Mushroom Pot Roast

This aromatic recipe is a nice change from traditional roasts. The creamy sauce uses no roux and is made right in the pot after the roast cooks. The savory sauce over the succulent roast is both elegant and appetizing without any of the fuss.

- **Hands-on time:** 10 minutes
- **Cook time:** 90 minutes

Serves 6

1 cup sliced button mushrooms

½ medium onion, sliced

1 tablespoon coconut oil

2 teaspoons dried minced onion

2 teaspoons dried parsley

1 teaspoon pepper

1 teaspoon garlic powder

½ teaspoon dried oregano

1 teaspoon salt

1 (2–3-pound) chuck roast

1 cup Beef Broth (see recipe in Chapter 3)

4 tablespoons butter

2 ounces cream cheese

¼ cup heavy cream

1 Press the Sauté button and add mushrooms, onion, and coconut oil to Instant Pot®. Stir-fry for 5 minutes or until onions turn translucent. While stir-frying, mix dried minced onion, parsley, pepper, garlic, oregano, and salt in small bowl. Rub into chuck roast.

2 Press the Cancel button. Add Beef Broth and roast into pot. Place butter and cream cheese on top. Click lid closed. Press the Meat button and press the Adjust button to set heat to More. Set time to 90 minutes.

3 When timer beeps allow a full natural release to retain moisture in meat. When pressure valve drops, stir in heavy cream. Remove roast carefully; it will be fall-apart tender. Press the Sauté button and reduce sauce in Instant Pot® for 10 minutes, stirring occasionally. Press the Cancel button and spoon over roast to serve.

CALORIES: 413

PROTEIN: 43.5 grams

FIBER: 0.6 grams

NET CARBOHYDRATES: 2.5 grams

FAT: 22.4 grams

SODIUM: 569 milligrams

CARBOHYDRATES: 3.1 grams

SUGAR: 1.4 grams

Salisbury Steak in Mushroom Sauce

This meal is filling and hearty after a long day, but won't set you back on your keto goals. Paired with cauliflower mash and green beans, this is a winning meal.

- **Hands-on time:** 10 minutes
- **Cook time:** 15 minutes

Serves 4

1 pound 85% lean ground beef
1 teaspoon steak seasoning
1 egg
2 tablespoons butter
½ medium onion, thinly sliced
½ cup sliced button mushrooms
1 cup Beef Broth (see recipe in Chapter 3)
2 ounces cream cheese
¼ cup heavy cream
¼ teaspoon xanthan gum

1 In large bowl mix ground beef, steak seasoning, and egg. Form 4 patties and set aside.

2 Press the Sauté button and add butter, onion, and mushrooms to Instant Pot®. Sauté 3–5 minutes or until onions are translucent and fragrant. Press the Cancel button.

3 Add broth, beef patties, and cream cheese to Instant Pot®. Click lid closed. Press the Manual button and adjust time for 15 minutes.

4 When timer beeps, allow a 10-minute natural release. Quick-release the remaining pressure. Carefully remove patties and set aside. Add heavy cream and xanthan gum. Whisk until fully mixed. Press the Sauté button and reduce gravy until desired thickness, about 5–10 minutes. Press the Cancel button and add patties back to Instant Pot® until ready to serve.

CALORIES: 420
PROTEIN: 24.6 grams
FIBER: 0.6 grams
NET CARBOHYDRATES: 2.4 grams

FAT: 30.5 grams
SODIUM: 323 milligrams
CARBOHYDRATES: 3.0 grams
SUGAR: 1.7 grams

Steak Bites and Roasted Garlic Dipping Sauce

Steak bites are a great light dish for when you want more than a snack, but less than a meal. An excellent source of protein and juicy flavor, these bites are quick to cook, and very quick to eat if you're not too careful!

- **Hands-on time: 5 minutes**
- **Cook time: 10 minutes**

Serves 4

Steak Bites

1 pound sirloin steak
1 teaspoon salt
¼ teaspoon pepper
4 tablespoons butter

Dipping Sauce

½ cup mayo
1 teaspoon lemon juice
1 roasted garlic clove, mashed
⅛ teaspoon red pepper flakes

1 Cut steak into 1-inch cubes. Sprinkle with salt and pepper. Press the Sauté button and add butter to Instant Pot®. When butter is melted, add steak and sear each side until desired doneness, about 10 minutes. Press the Cancel button and place steak bites into dish.

2 In medium bowl, mix mayo, lemon juice, roasted garlic, and red pepper flakes. Serve steak bites with dipping sauce.

CALORIES: 518	FAT: 43.4 grams
PROTEIN: 23.5 grams	SODIUM: 816 milligrams
FIBER: 0.1 grams	CARBOHYDRATES: 0.6 grams
NET CARBOHYDRATES: 0.5 grams	SUGAR: 0.2 grams

Bolognese Sauce

Even if you're nixing the pasta, you can still enjoy Italian favorites on the keto diet. This Bolognese is one low-carb sauce you should always have on hand for quick and tasty meals! Pair with spaghetti squash or zoodles.

- **Hands-on time:** 5 minutes
- **Cook time:** 10 minutes

Serves 4

1 pound 85% lean ground beef
2 cups Easy Tomato Sauce (see recipe in Chapter 4)

Place all ingredients into Instant Pot®. Click lid closed. Press the Manual button and adjust time for 10 minutes. When timer beeps, quick-release the pressure. Serve warm.

CALORIES: 373	**FAT:** 21.5 grams
PROTEIN: 24.9 grams	**SODIUM:** 614 milligrams
FIBER: 3.0 grams	**CARBOHYDRATES:** 14.4 grams
NET CARBOHYDRATES: 11.4 grams	**SUGAR:** 8.8 grams

Quick Bratwurst

You can enjoy a hot, juicy, perfectly cooked ballpark-style bratwurst at home, thanks to your Instant Pot®! No bun, no problem, for this low-carb dish.

- **Hands-on time:** 1 minute
- **Cook time:** 8 minutes

Serves 4

1 cup water
4 (4-ounce) bratwursts
1 tablespoon coconut oil

1 Pour water into Instant Pot® and place steam rack in bottom of pot. Put brats on steam rack and click lid closed. Adjust time for 10 minutes. When timer beeps, quick-release the pressure. Remove brats and pour out water.

2 Replace inner pot and press the Sauté button. Place brats and coconut oil into Instant Pot®. Brown for 2–4 minutes or until golden. Remove brats with tongs when golden. Serve alone or with buttered cabbage.

CALORIES: 312	**FAT:** 26.4 grams
PROTEIN: 11.7 grams	**SODIUM:** 719 milligrams
FIBER: 0.0 grams	**CARBOHYDRATES:** 2.4 grams
NET CARBOHYDRATES: 2.4 grams	**SUGAR:** 0.0 grams

Leftover Brisket Loaded Cauliflower Bowl

This Leftover Brisket Loaded Cauliflower Bowl is a hearty dish that will remind you of a baked potato! It's stuffed with all the tasty fixings you're used to, and even has a kick to it. Feel free to reduce or omit the jalapeños if you like a milder taste. You might want to add a dollop of sour cream to complete the ensemble.

- **Hands-on time:** 5 minutes
- **Cook time:** 15 minutes

Serves 4

1 cup water

2 cups fresh cauliflower, chopped into bite-sized pieces

3 tablespoons butter

¼ onion, diced

¼ cup pickled jalapeño slices

2 cups cooked brisket

2 ounces cream cheese, softened

1 cup shredded sharp cheddar cheese

¼ cup heavy cream

¼ cup cooked crumbled bacon

2 tablespoons sliced green onions

1 Add water to Instant Pot®. Place steamer basket into pot and add cauliflower. Click lid closed.

2 Press the Steam button and adjust time for 1 minute. When timer beeps, quick-release the steam and remove steamer basket with cauliflower; set aside. Do not remove excess moisture from cauliflower. Carefully pick up inner pot—it may be hot—and pour out water. Then place back inside Instant Pot®.

3 Press the Sauté button and add butter, onion, and jalapeño slices. Sauté for 4 minutes. Add cooked brisket and cream cheese. Continue cooking for 2 minutes. Add sharp cheddar, heavy cream, and cauliflower. Press the Cancel button.

4 Gently fold mixture until all ingredients are incorporated and cheese has melted. Sprinkle with crumbled bacon and green onions. Serve warm.

CALORIES: 574	**FAT:** 40.4 grams
PROTEIN: 32.7 grams	**SODIUM:** 557 milligrams
FIBER: 1.7 grams	**CARBOHYDRATES:** 9.6 grams
NET CARBOHYDRATES: 7.9 grams	**SUGAR:** 6.3 grams

Pork Chops in Mushroom Gravy

This easy dish feels elegant with the gravy atop it. Serve it alongside buttery green beans or a side salad with an oil-based dressing.

- **Hands-on time: 5 minutes**
- **Cook time: 15 minutes**

Serves 4

4 (5-ounce) pork chops
1 teaspoon salt
½ teaspoon pepper
2 tablespoons avocado oil
1 cup chopped button mushrooms
½ medium onion, sliced
1 clove garlic, minced
1 cup Chicken Broth (see recipe in Chapter 3)
¼ cup heavy cream
4 tablespoons butter
¼ teaspoon xanthan gum
1 tablespoon chopped fresh parsley

FREEZE IT!

Place in vacuum-sealed bag in the freezer for a quick last-minute meal!

1 Sprinkle pork chops with salt and pepper. Place avocado oil and mushrooms in Instant Pot® and press the Sauté button. Sauté 3–5 minutes until mushrooms begin to soften. Add onions and pork chops. Sauté additional 3 minutes until pork chops reach a golden brown.

2 Add garlic and broth to Instant Pot®. Click lid closed. Press the Manual button and adjust time for 15 minutes. When timer beeps, allow a 10-minute natural release. Quick-release the remaining pressure.

3 Remove lid and place pork chops on plate. Press the Sauté button and add heavy cream, butter, and xanthan gum. Reduce for 5–10 minutes or until sauce begins to thicken. Add pork chops back into pot. Serve warm topped with mushroom sauce and parsley.

CALORIES: 516
PROTEIN: 31.6 grams
FIBER: 0.8 grams
NET CARBOHYDRATES: 2.3 grams

FAT: 39.7 grams
SODIUM: 708 milligrams
CARBOHYDRATES: 3.1 grams
SUGAR: 1.4 grams

Spaghetti Squash Casserole

Ready to bring an Italian favorite into the low-carb world? This Spaghetti Squash Casserole puts together all of the rich flavors you're used to so well, you won't even miss the noodles. For an equally yummy vegetarian version, simply leave out the beef!

- **Hands-on time:** 10 minutes
- **Cook time:** 20 minutes

Serves 4

- 1 (6-pound) spaghetti squash, cooked
- 1 cup Easy Tomato Sauce (see recipe in Chapter 4)
- ½ cup whole-milk ricotta
- ¼ cup grated Parmesan cheese
- 3 tablespoons butter
- ½ teaspoon dried parsley
- ½ teaspoon garlic powder
- ¼ teaspoon dried basil
- ½ teaspoon salt
- ¼ teaspoon pepper
- 1 pound 85% lean ground beef, cooked
- 1 cup shredded whole-milk mozzarella cheese, divided
- 1 cup water

1 Use fork to scrape out inside of squash into long strands and place in 7-cup glass. Add remaining ingredients except for water, reserving half of mozzarella. Pour mixture into bowl. Sprinkle remaining cheese on top. Cover with foil.

2 Pour water into Instant Pot® and place steam rack on bottom. Place bowl on steam rack. Click lid closed. Press the Manual button and adjust time for 10 minutes. When timer beeps, natural-release the pressure. For a browned top, place dish in the oven under the broiler for a few minutes. Serve warm.

CALORIES: 628	FAT: 37.6 grams
PROTEIN: 36.5 grams	SODIUM: 1,002 milligrams
FIBER: 5.6 grams	CARBOHYDRATES: 28.6 grams
NET CARBOHYDRATES: 23 grams	SUGAR: 12.1 grams

Cabbage Egg Roll

If you've been missing egg rolls on your keto diet, you can find all their flavor in this dish. Of course, these won't have the crunchy exterior, but all the savory filling inside will make up for it. You can dip these in your favorite sauce or eat them alone. They're sure to be a hit!

- **Hands-on time:** 15 minutes
- **Cook time:** 5 minutes

Serves 4

1 pound 84% lean ground pork
2 tablespoons soy sauce
½ teaspoon salt
½ cup diced onion
1 clove garlic, minced
2 stalks green onion, sliced
8 cabbage leaves
1 cup water

1 Press the Sauté button and add ground pork, soy sauce, and salt to Instant Pot®. Brown pork until no pink remains. Carefully drain grease.

2 Add diced onion and continue cooking until translucent, 2–4 minutes. Add garlic and cook for additional 30 seconds. Press the Cancel button.

3 Pour mixture into large bowl; set aside. Mix green onions into pork. Rinse pot and replace. Add water and steam rack.

4 Take 2–3 tablespoons of pork mixture and spoon it into cabbage leaf in rectangle shape, off to one side of the leaf. Fold the short ends of the leaf toward the middle. Complete the roll by starting at the filled edge and rolling toward the empty side, as you would a burrito.

5 Place rolls onto steam rack. Click lid closed. Press the Manual button and adjust time for 1 minute. When timer beeps, quick-release the steam. Serve warm.

CALORIES: 257
PROTEIN: 22.5 grams
FIBER: 1.6 grams
NET CARBOHYDRATES: 3.8 grams

FAT: 15.9 grams
SODIUM: 807 milligrams
CARBOHYDRATES: 5.4 grams
SUGAR: 2.4 grams

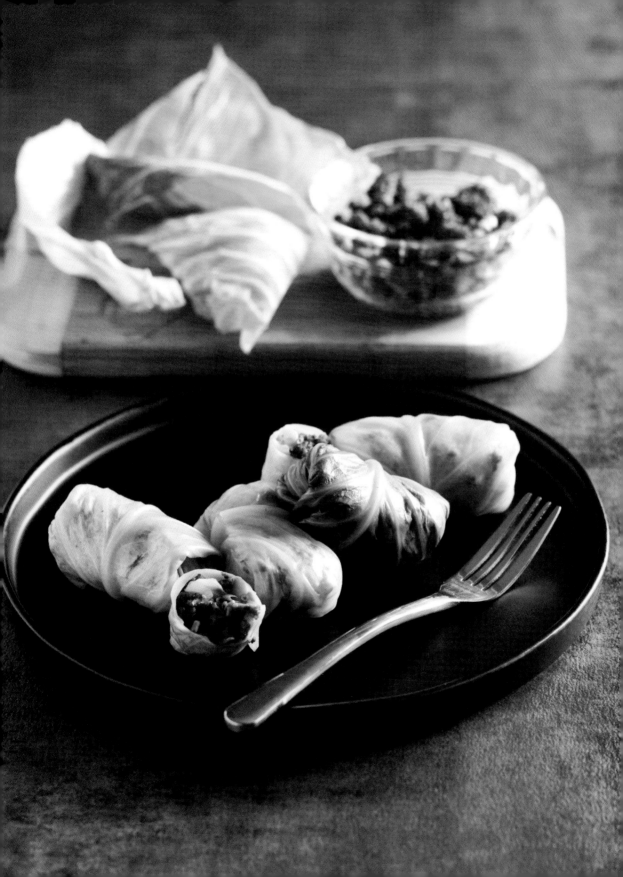

Mini BBQ Meatloaf

This Mini BBQ Meatloaf is a classic entrée you can count on to please the whole crowd. The tasty BBQ flavor is the icing on the cake here. Add a side of garlic cauliflower mash for a filling meal.

- **Hands-on time: 5 minutes**
- **Cook time: 25 minutes**

Serves 4

1 pound 85% lean ground beef

½ medium onion, diced

½ green pepper, diced

¼ cup almond flour

¼ cup shredded whole-milk mozzarella cheese

1 egg

1 teaspoon salt

¼ teaspoon pepper

1 teaspoon garlic powder

¼ cup Barbecue Sauce (see recipe in Chapter 5)

1 Mix all ingredients except barbecue sauce in large mixing bowl. Form into two small loaves and place into two (4-inch) loaf pans. Pour barbecue sauce on top of pans and cover with foil.

2 Pour water into Instant Pot® and place steam rack in bottom. Place one or both meatloaf pans on steam rack, depending on the size of your Instant Pot®, and click lid closed. Press the Manual button and adjust time to 25 minutes. When timer beeps, quick-release pressure.

CALORIES: 340

PROTEIN: 26.4 grams

FIBER: 1.5 grams

NET CARBOHYDRATES: 4.2 grams

FAT: 20.3 grams

SODIUM: 851 milligrams

CARBOHYDRATES: 5.6 grams

SUGAR: 1.8 grams

Easy BBQ Ribs

Ribs can be intimidating. We've all tasted delicious ribs, but it's much more rare to have cooked them yourself. Especially since they're meant to be shared, you want them to be mouthwateringly juicy, and fall-off-the-bone tender. These fit the bill. Plus, this recipe is so easy, you'll want to add them to your weekly rotation!

- **Hands-on time: 5 minutes**
- **Cook time: 50 minutes**

Serves 4

1 (4-pound) rack ribs
1 tablespoon chili powder
1 teaspoon salt
1 teaspoon dried parsley
½ teaspoon pepper
½ teaspoon garlic powder
½ teaspoon onion powder
½ cup Barbecue Sauce (see recipe in Chapter 5), divided
1 cup water
1 tablespoon liquid smoke

BROIL IT!

For a caramelized sauce, broil in oven for 3–5 minutes, watching carefully so it does not burn.

1 Remove the membrane on the underside of the ribs by running a knife under the rack. Rub ribs with seasonings and half barbecue sauce.

2 Place steam rack into Instant Pot® and pour in water and liquid smoke. Place rack on steam rack and click lid closed. Press the Meat button and press the Adjust button to set heat to More for fall-off-the-bone ribs. Set timer for 50 minutes.

3 When timer beeps, place ribs on foil-lined baking sheet and brush with remaining sauce.

CALORIES: 421
PROTEIN: 39.5 grams
FIBER: 1.3 grams
NET CARBOHYDRATES: 3.5 grams

FAT: 23.6 grams
SODIUM: 990 milligrams
CARBOHYDRATES: 4.8 grams
SUGAR: 1.2 grams

Cheesy Beef and Broccoli

This is an especially satisfying last-minute meal. It doesn't take long to cook and freezes well too. It's a true comfort food that's very filling even though it has only a few ingredients. This is also great for your low-carb weekly meal prep because you can easily double the batch and separate into containers for the week.

- **Hands-on time: 5 minutes**
- **Cook time: 10 minutes**

Serves 4

1 pound 85% lean ground beef

1 teaspoon salt

½ teaspoon garlic powder

½ teaspoon dried parsley

¼ teaspoon dried oregano

2 tablespoons butter

¾ cup Beef Broth (see recipe in Chapter 3)

2 cups broccoli florets

¼ cup heavy cream

1 cup shredded mild cheddar cheese

1 Press the Sauté button and brown ground beef in Instant Pot® until there's no more pink. Press the Cancel button. Sprinkle seasonings over meat and add butter, broth, and broccoli. Click lid closed.

2 Press the Manual button and set time for 2 minutes. When timer beeps, press the Cancel button. Stir in heavy cream and cheddar until completely melted.

CALORIES: 476	FAT: 33.5 grams
PROTEIN: 29.9 grams	SODIUM: 860 milligrams
FIBER: 1.3 grams	CARBOHYDRATES: 4.3 grams
NET CARBOHYDRATES: 3.0 grams	SUGAR: 1.3 grams

Taco Cabbage Casserole

This is the perfect one-pot meal when you're short on time. Loaded with taco flavor, the cabbage in this recipe gives the dish a nutritious boost that helps fill you up while offering a yummy crunch! Not a big fan of spice? Top your portion with a dollop of sour cream to help cut the heat from the chili powder.

- **Hands-on time: 5 minutes**
- **Cook time: 4 minutes**

Serves 4

1 pound 85% lean ground beef

2 cups shredded white cabbage

1 cup salsa

1 teaspoon salt

1 tablespoon chili powder

½ teaspoon cumin

½ cup water

1 cup shredded cheddar cheese

1 Press the Sauté button and brown ground beef. Once fully cooked, add remaining ingredients except for cheese.

2 Click lid closed. Press the Manual button and adjust timer for 4 minutes. When timer beeps, quick-release the pressure and stir in cheddar.

CALORIES: 393	FAT: 23.0 grams
PROTEIN: 29.5 grams	SODIUM: 1,148 milligrams
FIBER: 2.4 grams	CARBOHYDRATES: 7.5 grams
NET CARBOHYDRATES: 5.1 grams	SUGAR: 1.4 grams

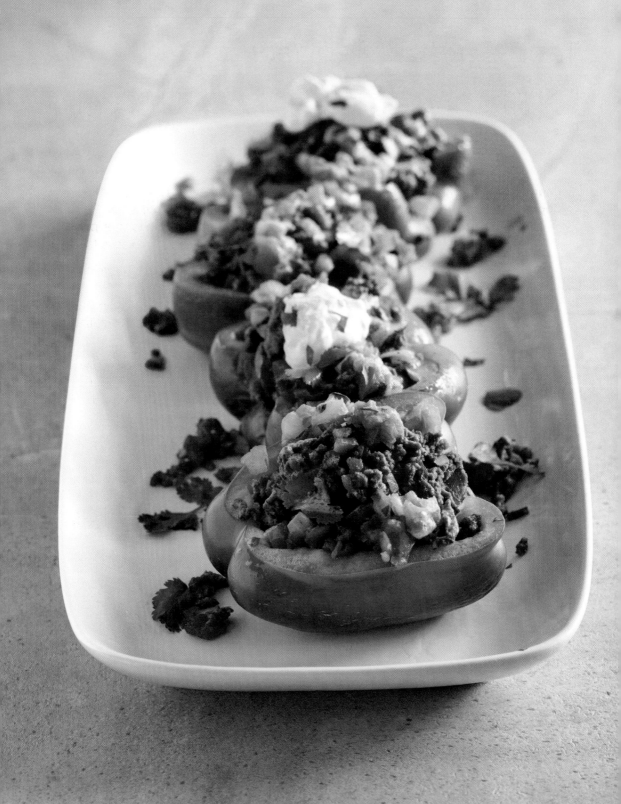

Taco Stuffed Peppers

These peppers are super easy to make, and are done in a fraction of the time it takes to cook traditional stuffed peppers. You certainly won't miss the rice in this recipe, especially once you add your favorite toppings. This is a meal you can get on the table in under 30 minutes—and the whole family will enjoy.

- **Hands-on time: 5 minutes**
- **Cook time: 10 minutes**

Serves 6

1 pound 85% lean ground beef

¼ cup diced tomatoes and green chilies

¼ cup diced onion

1 teaspoon salt

1 teaspoon chili powder

1 teaspoon cumin

1 cup water

6 green bell peppers cut in half lengthwise, seeds removed

Toppings such as salsa, sour cream, chopped cilantro, chopped red onion, and so on (not included in nutritional analysis)

1 Press the Sauté button and place ground beef into Instant Pot®. Break into small pieces and cook until beef is no longer pink. Carefully drain grease if there is excess fat.

2 Replace pot and add tomatoes and chilies, onion, salt, chili powder, and cumin. Mix ingredients until fully combined. Spoon mixture into pepper halves and rinse pot with water.

3 Replace pot and add water. Place steamer basket into pot and carefully add pepper halves. Click lid closed. Press the Manual button and adjust timer for 4 minutes.

4 When timer beeps, quick-release the pressure and add favorite toppings to serve.

CALORIES: 139
PROTEIN: 12.8 grams
FIBER: 2.6 grams
NET CARBOHYDRATES: 4.5 grams

FAT: 5.8 grams
SODIUM: 467 milligrams
CARBOHYDRATES: 7.1 grams
SUGAR: 3.5 grams

Butter Beef and Spinach

Meal prep for the week couldn't be easier with this dish. It's simple but loaded with fat to keep you full. You can dress it up or down with salsa, avocado, and your favorite sauce, or just keep it simple as is. It's easy to double the recipe and freeze for those busy weeknights.

- **Hands-on time:** 2 minutes
- **Cook time:** 10 minutes

Serves 4

1 pound 85% lean ground beef
1 cup water
4 cups fresh spinach
¾ teaspoon salt
¼ cup butter
¼ teaspoon pepper
¼ teaspoon garlic powder

1 Press the Sauté button and add ground beef to Instant Pot®. Brown beef until fully cooked and spoon into 7-cup glass bowl. Drain grease and replace pot.

2 Pour water into pot and place steam rack in bottom. Place baking dish on steam rack and add fresh spinach, salt, butter, pepper, and garlic powder to ground beef. Cover with aluminum foil. Click lid closed.

3 Press the Manual button and adjust time for 2 minutes. When timer beeps, quick-release the pressure. Remove aluminum foil and stir.

CALORIES: 272
PROTEIN: 18.3 grams
FIBER: 0.7 grams
NET CARBOHYDRATES: 0.6 grams

FAT: 19.1 grams
SODIUM: 516 milligrams
CARBOHYDRATES: 1.3 grams
SUGAR: 0.1 grams

Pizza Casserole

Perhaps the dish people miss the most after going low-carb is pizza, but it's not the crust that makes pizza one of America's favorite foods…it's the toppings! And the toppings are all keto-friendly! This casserole shows you how to achieve the same pizza taste you're used to in a creamy bowl. The flavors are so savory, you won't even miss the crust! Feel free to adjust toppings and amounts to your liking. Customize this casserole any way you like, but keep in mind that your changes will affect the nutritional information.

- **Hands-on time:** 10 minutes
- **Cook time:** 15 minutes

Serves 4

½ pound Italian sausage
¼ cup diced onion
¼ cup diced green pepper
¼ cup cooked bacon crumbles
16 slices pepperoni
2 cups shredded whole-milk mozzarella cheese
2 cups fresh spinach
1½ cups Easy Tomato Sauce (see recipe in Chapter 4)
½ cup grated Parmesan cheese

1 Press the Sauté button and add sausage to Instant Pot®. Brown until no pink remains. Add onion, pepper, and bacon crumbles. Continue cooking until onion softens.

2 Gently fold remaining ingredients except Parmesan into Instant Pot®. Sprinkle with Parmesan. Serve warm.

CALORIES: 616
PROTEIN: 33.3 grams
FIBER: 2.9 grams
NET CARBOHYDRATES: 13.3 grams

FAT: 43.4 grams
SODIUM: 1,742 milligrams
CARBOHYDRATES: 16.2 grams
SUGAR: 7.9 grams

Cheeseburger Casserole

This is a family-friendly meal that will have the kids coming back for more. Let this recipe act as a base and add your own favorite ingredients. You may be surprised that even a little lettuce on top can really make it taste like a burger, but without the carbs.

- **Hands-on time:** 5 minutes
- **Cook time:** 15 minutes

Serves 4

1 pound 85% lean ground beef
½ teaspoon salt
¼ teaspoon pepper
¼ teaspoon garlic powder
2 tablespoons butter
¼ cup diced onion
¼ cup mayo
1 teaspoon yellow mustard
1 tablespoon tomato paste
1 egg
1 cup shredded cheddar cheese, divided

1 Press the Sauté button and add ground beef to Instant Pot®. Brown meat until fully cooked. Add salt, pepper, garlic powder, butter, and onion to pot. Sauté until onions are translucent. Press the Cancel button.

2 Spoon meat mixture into 7-cup glass bowl and add mayo, mustard, tomato paste, egg, and ½ cup of cheddar. Mix well. Top with remaining cheddar. Cover with aluminum foil.

3 Pour water into Instant Pot® and add steam rack. Set bowl on steam rack. Click lid closed. Press the Manual button and adjust time for 15 minutes. When timer beeps, quick-release the pressure.

CALORIES: 442
PROTEIN: 29.8 grams
FIBER: 0.4 grams
NET CARBOHYDRATES: 2.0 grams
FAT: 29.8 grams
SODIUM: 575 milligrams
CARBOHYDRATES: 2.4 grams
SUGAR: 1.1 grams

Burger Bowl

Deliciously juicy steamed cheeseburgers can be ready in minutes thanks to your Instant Pot®. Steaming burgers might not be the most popular method of cooking them, but with this recipe you'll wonder how you didn't discover it sooner.

- **Hands-on time:** 15 minutes
- **Cook time:** 10 minutes

Serves 4

1 pound 85% lean ground beef
½ teaspoon salt
¼ teaspoon pepper
½ medium onion, sliced
2 cups shredded lettuce
1 cup shredded cheddar cheese
4 pickle spears
1 avocado, sliced

1 Press the Sauté button and add ground beef to Instant Pot®. When meat is browned completely, drain if needed.

2 Add salt, pepper, and onion. Continue cooking until onion is soft and translucent. Press the Cancel button.

3 Divide lettuce into four sections. Top each section with a quarter of the ground beef. Add a quarter of the cheddar, one pickle spear, and sliced avocado. Top with favorite sauce or dressing.

CALORIES: 429
PROTEIN: 29.2 grams
FIBER: 3.4 grams
NET CARBOHYDRATES: 3.2 grams

FAT: 27.3 grams
SODIUM: 836 milligrams
CARBOHYDRATES: 6.6 grams
SUGAR: 1.9 grams

Layered Zucchini Lasagna

Italian foods can be tricky to replace after cutting the carbs because pasta is such a huge part of Italian cuisine. Luckily, if you focus on getting the other flavors and seasonings just right, you won't even miss the pasta. Even better, this recipe has all the right proportions to make this lasagna a weekly favorite!

- **Hands-on time:** 20 minutes
- **Cook time:** 5 minutes

Serves 4

½ pound 85% lean ground beef

½ pound 84% lean ground pork

½ medium onion, diced

1 cup Easy Tomato Sauce (see recipe in Chapter 4)

4 zucchini, cut into long slices

½ cup whole-milk ricotta

¼ cup grated Parmesan cheese

1 cup shredded whole-milk mozzarella cheese, divided

½ teaspoon salt

¼ teaspoon garlic powder

¼ teaspoon dried oregano

¼ teaspoon dried parsley

1 cup water

1. Press the Sauté button and add beef, pork, and onion to Instant Pot®. Brown meat until no pink remains. While meat is browning, prepare zucchini and filling.

2. Place zucchini slices in single layer between paper towels and set aside.

3. In medium bowl, mix ricotta, Parmesan, half of mozzarella, and seasonings. Set aside.

4. When meat is completely cooked, spoon into a separate medium bowl and prepare to assemble lasagna. Place layer of zucchini strips on bottom of 7-inch springform pan or cake pan. Spoon ⅓ of meat onto strips and spread evenly. Spoon ½ of cheese mixture and tomato sauce onto meat layer.

5. Complete next layer of zucchini, meat, cheese, and tomato sauce. For third layer, top meat with remaining mozzarella. Cover with foil.

6. Pour water into Instant Pot® and place steam rack in bottom. Place covered pan onto steam rack and click lid closed. Press the Manual button and adjust time for 5 minutes. When timer beeps, quick-release the pressure. Serve warm with salad and high-fat dressing.

CALORIES: 513

PROTEIN: 36.7 grams

FIBER: 3.8 grams

NET CARBOHYDRATES: 13.7 grams

FAT: 29.9 grams

SODIUM: 966 milligrams

CARBOHYDRATES: 17.5 grams

SUGAR: 10.3 grams

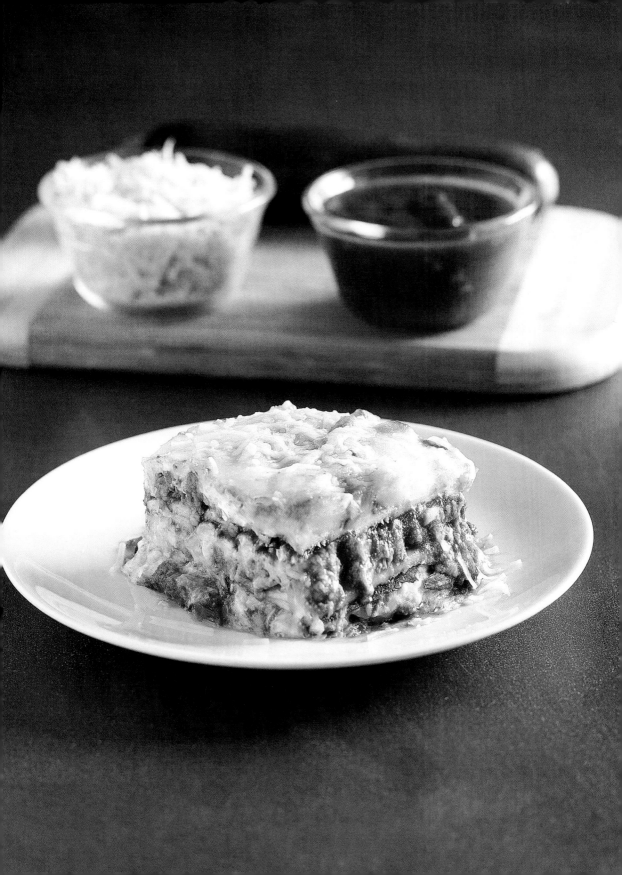

Sloppy Joes

This dish will take you right back to grade school cafeteria lunch! Not only is it kid-friendly, it's keto-friendly too. Of course you'll ditch the bun, so you can serve them in lettuce wraps for added nutrition.

- **Hands-on time:** 10 minutes
- **Cook time:** 10 minutes

Serves 4

1 pound 85% lean ground beef

½ green pepper, diced

½ medium onion, diced

3 tablespoons tomato paste

1 tablespoon erythritol

½ teaspoon yellow mustard

½ cup Beef Broth (see recipe in Chapter 3)

1 teaspoon salt

½ teaspoon garlic powder

⅛ teaspoon pepper

1 Press the Sauté button and brown ground beef in Instant Pot®. When no pink remains, add in remaining ingredients.

2 Stir frequently and reduce liquid until desired consistency. Serve warm.

CALORIES: 263
PROTEIN: 22.2 grams
FIBER: 1.2 grams
NET CARBOHYDRATES: 3.5 grams
SUGAR ALCOHOLS: 3.0 grams

FAT: 14.6 grams
SODIUM: 671 milligrams
CARBOHYDRATES: 7.7 grams
SUGAR: 2.4 grams

8

Seafood and Fish Main Dishes

Fish is one of the most intimidating types of cuisine to prepare, even for those who really know their way around the kitchen. All types of seafood are desirable for a keto diet, especially because of their amazing flavor and countless health benefits, but fish recipes can be pretty daunting.

Enter the Instant Pot®. This device is perfect for creating fresh and flavorful fish and seafood recipes! Your Instant Pot® can steam up any fish dish in minutes, locking in the nutrients and all the fresh taste. Fish like salmon and tuna, as well as seafood like shrimp and crab, are all sources of omega-3 fatty acids, which are important for maintaining a healthy and effective metabolism.

The quick-release recipes in this chapter will make you feel like a master of seafood. From Crispy Blackened Salmon to Snow Crab Legs with Butter Sauce, you'll be ready to try new dishes that will become family favorites in no time!

Snow Crab Legs with Butter Sauce

Make sure you have a seafood cracker handy...these snow crab legs aren't going to crack themselves! But they will steam up beautifully in just minutes using your Instant Pot®. Serve them with melted butter and a generous spritz of lemon to enhance the crustaceous flavor.

- **Hands-on time:** 3 minutes
- **Cook time:** 7 minutes

Serves 2

2 pounds crab legs
1 cup water
4 tablespoons butter
1 garlic clove, finely minced
½ lemon, juiced
4 lemon wedges

1 Rinse crab legs. Pour water into Instant Pot®. Place steamer basket and crab legs into Instant Pot®. Click lid closed. Press the Steam button and adjust time for 7 minutes. When timer beeps, quick-release the pressure. Crab legs will be bright pink when done.

2 In small bowl, melt butter and add garlic.

3 Squeeze lemon juice into butter or over legs and crack legs open. Serve with butter sauce and lemon wedges.

CALORIES: 511
PROTEIN: 66.7 grams
FIBER: 0.1 grams
NET CARBOHYDRATES: 0.9 grams

FAT: 22.5 grams
SODIUM: 3,036 milligrams
CARBOHYDRATES: 1.0 grams
SUGAR: 0.2 grams

Shrimp and Crab Stew

This hearty stew is packed with flavor and two kinds of seafood. Feel free to add extra meat—whatever is fresh at the market will be a wonderful addition.

- **Hands-on time:** 10 minutes
- **Cook time:** 15 minutes

Serves 4

1 tablespoon coconut oil

½ medium onion, diced

2 cloves garlic, minced

2 stalks celery, chopped

1 bay leaf

2 teaspoons Old Bay seasoning

1 teaspoon salt

1 pound shrimp, shelled, deveined, and chopped

1 pound lump crab meat

4 cups Seafood Stock (see recipe in Chapter 3)

2 tablespoons butter

¼ cup heavy cream

1 Press the Sauté button and add coconut oil to Instant Pot®. Sauté onions for 3 minutes or until translucent. Add garlic and sauté 30 seconds. Press the Cancel button.

2 Add all remaining ingredients except heavy cream. Click lid closed.

3 Press the Manual button and adjust time for 10 minutes. When timer beeps, quick-release the pressure. Stir in heavy cream. Serve warm.

CALORIES: 326	FAT: 15.4 grams
PROTEIN: 28.3 grams	SODIUM: 2,048 milligrams
FIBER: 0.8 grams	CARBOHYDRATES: 4.0 grams
NET CARBOHYDRATES: 3.2 grams	SUGAR: 1.4 grams

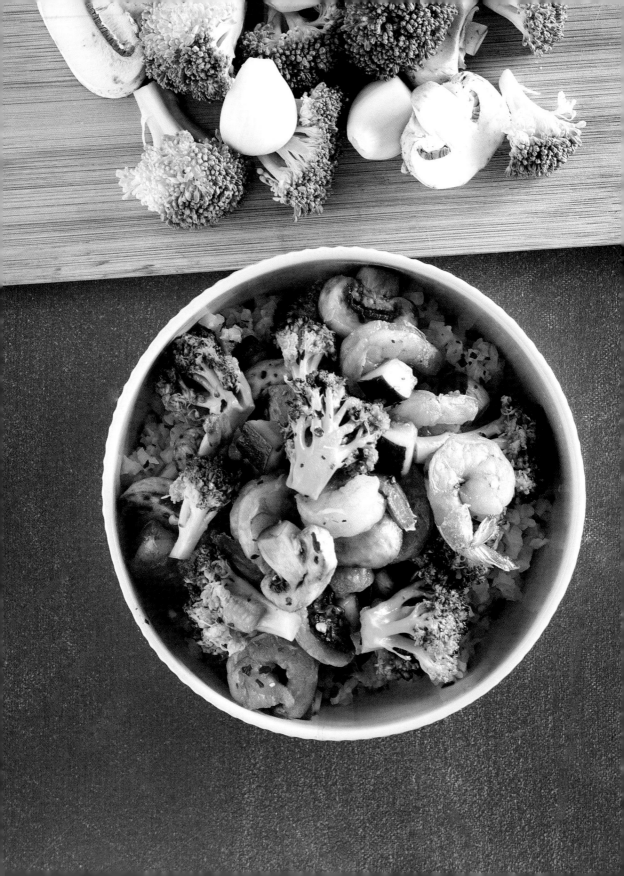

Shrimp Stir-Fry

Shrimp's mild flavor can handle almost any flavor profile and it cooks in the blink of an eye. If you're used to buying precooked shrimp, I encourage you to learn how to devein and shell your own shrimp—the flavor is worlds apart! This stir-fry works with either kind and is still just as delicious. Feel free to add more veggies and spice it up to suit your tastes!

- **Hands-on time: 10 minutes**
- **Cook time: 10 minutes**

Serves 4

2 tablespoons coconut oil

1 pound medium shrimp, shelled and deveined

½ cup button mushrooms

½ cup diced zucchini

2 cups broccoli florets

¼ cup soy sauce or liquid aminos

2 cloves garlic, minced

⅛ teaspoon red pepper flakes

2 cups cooked cauliflower rice

1 Press the Sauté button and add coconut oil to Instant Pot®. Add shrimp and cook for 5 minutes or until pink and fully cooked. Remove and set aside in bowl.

2 Add mushrooms, zucchini, broccoli, soy sauce, garlic, and red pepper flakes to pot. Stir-fry for 3–5 minutes until vegetables are fork-tender. Add shrimp back to pot and press Cancel.

3 Separate premade, warmed cauliflower rice into each bowl and top with portion of stir-fry. Serve warm.

CALORIES: 173

PROTEIN: 19.3 grams

FIBER: 1.4 grams

NET CARBOHYDRATES: 5.6 grams

FAT: 7.4 grams

SODIUM: 1,538 milligrams

CARBOHYDRATES: 7.0 grams

SUGAR: 1.6 grams

Easy Peel-and-Eat Shrimp

Shrimp is a great source of protein as well as the mineral selenium, which contains heart-healthy benefits like preventing coronary heart disease and fighting inflammation. Treat your body to an easy serving of these benefits with this simple dish.

- **Hands-on time:** 5 minutes
- **Cook time:** 3 minutes

Serves 4

2 pounds raw shell-on shrimp

1 cup Seafood Stock (see recipe in Chapter 3)

1 teaspoon Old Bay seasoning

1 Use a knife to cut slit in shell and devein shrimp while leaving rest of shell intact. Pour Seafood Stock and Old Bay seasoning into Instant Pot®. Add shrimp. Click lid closed.

2 Press the Manual button and set time for 3 minutes. When timer beeps, quick-release the pressure. To eat, remove shell and serve warm with low-carb cocktail sauce.

CALORIES: 81

PROTEIN: 15.7 grams

FIBER: 0.0 grams

NET CARBOHYDRATES: 1.0 grams

FAT: 0.8 grams

SODIUM: 671 milligrams

CARBOHYDRATES: 1.0 grams

SUGAR: 0.0 grams

Buttered Scallops

Scallops are a delicate and delicious dish. The secret is to get a great sear on the outside. Just be careful not to overcook them. These pair well with a crisp green salad or roasted veggies.

- **Hands-on time:** 5 minutes
- **Cook time:** 5 minutes

Serves 4

2 tablespoons avocado oil

1 pound large sea scallops

⅛ teaspoon salt

⅛ teaspoon pepper

2 tablespoons melted butter

1 Press the Sauté button and add avocado oil to Instant Pot®. Allow to fully preheat.

2 Remove side muscle from scallops. Pat dry with towel and sprinkle with salt and pepper. When Instant Pot® reads "hot," carefully add scallops to pan and sear for 2 minutes. Carefully turn and sear opposite side for 2–3 minutes. They will appear opaque all the way through when finished.

3 Pour butter over scallops and serve hot.

CALORIES: 190

PROTEIN: 13.7 grams

FIBER: 0.0 grams

NET CARBOHYDRATES: 3.7 grams

FAT: 12.4 grams

SODIUM: 517 milligrams

CARBOHYDRATES: 3.7 grams

SUGAR: 0.0 grams

Shrimp Scampi

Buttery and flavorful, this shrimp scampi is a weeknight staple. In under 10 minutes, this lemon cream sauce takes shape, so you'll have dinner on the table in no time.

- **Hands-on time: 10 minutes**
- **Cook time: 10 minutes**

Serves 4

4 tablespoons butter

2 teaspoons finely minced garlic

1 pound shrimp, peeled and deveined

1 cup Chicken Broth (see recipe in Chapter 3)

1 tablespoon lemon juice

½ teaspoon salt

¼ cup heavy cream

¼ teaspoon xanthan gum

1 tablespoon chopped fresh parsley

¼ teaspoon red pepper flakes

1 Press the Sauté button and then press the Adjust button to set heat to Less. Add butter and garlic to pot and sauté 1–3 minutes until fragrant. Press the Cancel button.

2 Add shrimp, broth, lemon juice, and salt to Instant Pot®. Click lid closed. Press the Manual button and adjust time for 4 minutes.

3 When timer beeps, quick-release the pressure. Remove lid and stir in heavy cream and xanthan gum. Garnish with parsley and red pepper flakes.

CALORIES: 242

PROTEIN: 16.4 grams

FIBER: 0.3 grams

NET CARBOHYDRATES: 2.2 grams

FAT: 22.0 grams

SODIUM: 941 milligrams

CARBOHYDRATES: 2.5 grams

SUGAR: 0.6 grams

Lemon Dill Salmon

Lemon and dill are the most classic flavors to complement salmon. They're simple, yet when combined, really elevate the flavor of the fish and turn this easy meal into an elegant dinner. Pair with fresh spinach and a tablespoon of butter to complete the meal.

- **Hands-on time:** 3 minutes
- **Cook time:** 5 minutes

Serves 2

2 (1-inch-thick, 3-ounce) salmon filets
1 teaspoon chopped fresh dill
½ teaspoon salt
¼ teaspoon pepper
1 cup water
2 tablespoons lemon juice
½ lemon, sliced

1 Sprinkle salmon with dill, salt, and pepper. Place steam rack into Instant Pot® and pour water into pot. Place salmon on steam rack, skin side down. Squeeze lemon juice over filets and put lemon slices on top. Click lid closed.

2 Press the Steam button and adjust time to 5 minutes. When timer beeps, quick-release the pressure. Use meat thermometer to ensure fish has completely cooked to at least 145°F. Serve with additional dill and lemon slices.

CALORIES: 127
PROTEIN: 17.1 grams
FIBER: 0.3 grams
NET CARBOHYDRATES: 1.5 grams
FAT: 4.9 grams
SODIUM: 618 milligrams
CARBOHYDRATES: 1.8 grams
SUGAR: 0.4 grams

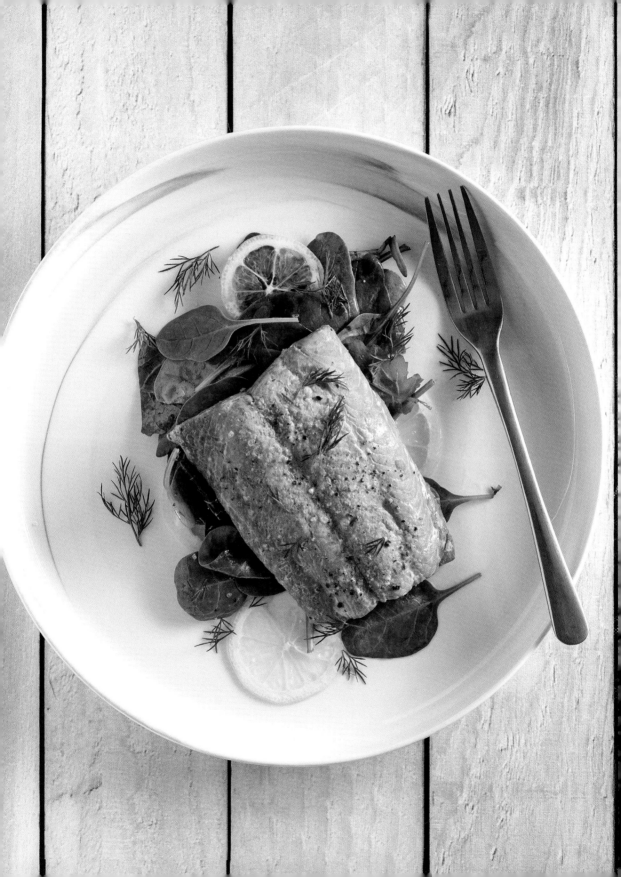

Lemon Butter Lobster Tail

Surf-and-turf meals just got easier. You can have fresh cooked lobster tail in no time in the Instant Pot®. You can sear a steak on the stovetop and steam lobster at the same time for a restaurant-quality meal that takes under 15 minutes!

- **Hands-on time: 5 minutes**
- **Cook time: 4 minutes**

Serves 2

1 cup Chicken Broth (see recipe in Chapter 3)
½ cup water
1 teaspoon Old Bay seasoning
2 (12-ounce) fresh lobster tails
Juice of ½ lemon
2 tablespoons butter, melted
¼ teaspoon salt
¼ teaspoon dried parsley
⅛ teaspoon pepper

1 Pour broth, water, and Old Bay seasoning into Instant Pot®. Place steam rack in bottom. Place lobster tails on steam rack, shell side down. Click lid closed.

2 Press the Manual button and adjust time for 4 minutes. When timer beeps, quick-release the pressure.

3 In small bowl, combine lemon juice, butter, salt, parsley, and pepper.

4 Crack open tail and dip into butter sauce.

CALORIES: 259
PROTEIN: 32.9 grams
FIBER: 0.1 grams
NET CARBOHYDRATES: 0.7 grams

FAT: 17.3 grams
SODIUM: 1,160 grams
CARBOHYDRATES: 0.8 grams
SUGAR: 0.3 grams

Lobster Mac 'n' Cheese

Try this twist on macaroni and cheese with all the flavor and a fraction of the carbs. The lobster is juicy and adds a nice sweet flavor to the gooey cheeses. It may sound crazy at first, but cauliflower makes a great pasta replacement. It is full of nutrients and really soaks up the flavor of the meal.

- **Hands-on time:** 10 minutes
- **Cook time:** 15 minutes

Serves 4

1 large head cauliflower, chopped into bite-sized pieces
1 cup water
4 tablespoons butter
½ medium onion, diced
4 ounces cream cheese
¼ cup heavy cream
½ cup grated Gruyère cheese
½ cup shredded sharp cheddar cheese
1 teaspoon hot sauce
1 teaspoon salt
½ teaspoon pepper
1 pound cooked lobster meat

FOR A CRISPY TOPPING

To get that classic mac 'n' cheese browned top, pour mixture into oven-safe baking dish and add crushed pork rinds to top. Broil for 3–5 minutes until pork rinds are golden and crispy.

1 Place cauliflower on steamer basket. Add water to Instant Pot® and place steamer basket in bottom of pot. Click lid closed. Press the Steam button and adjust time for 1 minute.

2 When timer beeps, quick-release the pressure and remove steamer basket. Set cauliflower aside. Pour water out of pot and wipe dry.

3 Replace pot and press the Sauté button. Press the Adjust button to set heat to Less. Add butter and onion. Sauté for 3–5 minutes or until onion becomes soft and fragrant. Soften cream cheese in microwave and stir with spoon until smooth. Add cream cheese to Instant Pot®. Press the Cancel button. Press the Sauté button and press the Adjust button to set heat to Normal.

4 Add heavy cream to pot and bring to simmer. Continuously stir until ingredients are fully incorporated. Press the Cancel button.

5 Add shredded cheeses and stir quickly to melt. Add cooked cauliflower into pot, stirring until fully coated with cheese. Add hot sauce and seasoning. Chop lobster into bite-sized pieces and fold into pot. Serve warm.

CALORIES: 521	**FAT:** 33.8 grams
PROTEIN: 35.3 grams	**SODIUM:** 1,500 milligrams
FIBER: 4.5 grams	**CARBOHYDRATES:** 13.7 grams
NET CARBOHYDRATES: 9.2 grams	**SUGAR:** 6.0 grams

Spicy Cream Shrimp

This is a dish that definitely bites back! If you love all things spicy, your taste buds will be happy to enjoy the fierce heat from this firecracker shrimp! Serve with broccoli as a mild side.

- **Hands-on time: 5 minutes**
- **Cook time: 7 minutes**

Serves 2

1 pound shrimp, peeled and deveined
½ teaspoon Old Bay seasoning
¼ teaspoon salt
¼ teaspoon pepper
⅛ teaspoon cayenne
⅛ teaspoon garlic powder
1 cup water
¼ cup mayo
2 tablespoons chili paste

1 Toss shrimp in 7-cup glass bowl with Old Bay seasoning, salt, pepper, cayenne, and garlic.

2 Pour water into Instant Pot®. Place steam rack into pot and place bowl with shrimp on top. Click lid closed and press the Steam button. Adjust time for 7 minutes.

3 When timer beeps, do a quick release and carefully remove bowl from Instant Pot®. Drain water. In small bowl, mix mayo and chili paste. Add to shrimp and toss to coat. Serve warm.

CALORIES: 399
PROTEIN: 32.2 grams
FIBER: 0.1 grams
NET CARBOHYDRATES: 8.5 grams

FAT: 24.3 grams
SODIUM: 2,259 milligrams
CARBOHYDRATES: 8.6 grams
SUGAR: 4.2 grams

Shrimp and Cauliflower Rice

This meal couldn't be easier. In less than 20 minutes, this meal can be cooked and on the table. It adapts to your seasoning preference and accommodates extra veggies. The cauliflower rice is filling but won't leave you with the carb bloat that white rice would.

- **Hands-on time: 3 minutes**
- **Cook time: 5 minutes**

Serves 2

1 pound shrimp, peeled and deveined
½ teaspoon salt
¼ teaspoon pepper
¼ teaspoon garlic powder
¼ teaspoon dried parsley
6 asparagus spears
1 cup water
2 tablespoons butter
1 cup uncooked cauliflower rice

1 Sprinkle seasoning on shrimp and place on steamer basket. Cut asparagus into bite-sized pieces and add to steamer basket.

2 Pour water into Instant Pot® and place steamer basket in bottom. Click lid closed. Press the Steam button and adjust time for 5 minutes.

3 When timer beeps, quick-release the pressure. Remove steamer basket and pour water out of Instant Pot®. Replace pot and press the Sauté button. Add butter to Instant Pot® along with cauliflower rice and cooked shrimp and asparagus. Stir-fry for 3–5 minutes until cauliflower is tender.

CALORIES: 283
PROTEIN: 33.1 grams
FIBER: 2.1 grams
NET CARBOHYDRATES: 4.3 grams

FAT: 12.4 grams
SODIUM: 1,876 milligrams
CARBOHYDRATES: 6.4 grams
SUGAR: 1.9 grams

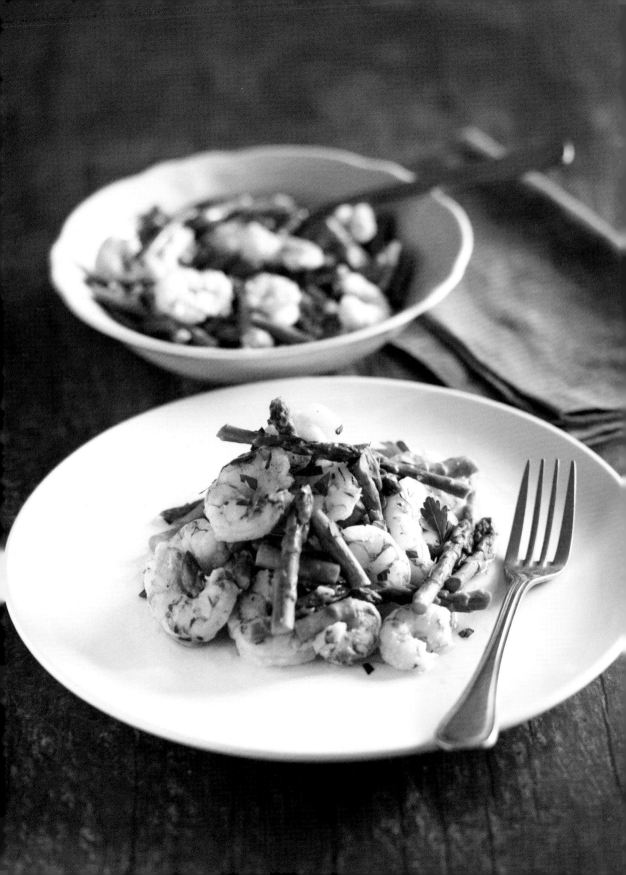

Garlic Butter Shrimp and Asparagus

This meal is a quick one that you can prepare even for lunch in no time. A hint of spice from the red peppers and an overall zest from the lemon juice pull this meal together.

- **Hands-on time: 5 minutes**
- **Cook time: 3 minutes**

Serves 2

1 pound uncooked peeled shrimp, deveined

1 clove garlic, finely minced

½ teaspoon salt

¼ teaspoon pepper

¼ teaspoon paprika

⅛ teaspoon red pepper flakes

½ pound asparagus, cut into bite-sized pieces

Juice of ½ lemon

4 tablespoons butter

2 teaspoons chopped fresh parsley

1 cup water

1 Sprinkle shrimp with garlic, salt, pepper, paprika, and red pepper flakes and place in 7-cup glass bowl. Place asparagus in bowl.

2 Squeeze lemon juice over shrimp and asparagus and gently mix. Cut butter into cubes and place around dish. Sprinkle with parsley. Cover with foil. Add water to Instant Pot® and place steam rack in bottom of pot. Carefully place dish on steam rack and click lid closed.

3 Press the Steam button and adjust time for 3 minutes. When timer beeps, quick-release the pressure. Remove dish from pot. Serve warm.

CALORIES: 381

PROTEIN: 32.7 grams

FIBER: 1.6 grams

NET CARBOHYDRATES: 4.3 grams

FAT: 23.2 grams

SODIUM: 1,868 milligrams

CARBOHYDRATES: 5.9 grams

SUGAR: 1.5 grams

Salmon Burger with Avocado

This dish combines two excellent fat sources into one simple meal. Avocado is packed with fiber, vitamins, and healthy fats. Salmon is an excellent source of omega-3s as well as vitamins that keep you healthy and energized.

- **Hands-on time:** 10 minutes
- **Cook time:** 5 minutes

Serves 4

2 tablespoons coconut oil
1 pound salmon filets
½ teaspoon salt
¼ teaspoon garlic powder
¼ teaspoon chili powder
2 tablespoons finely diced onion
1 egg
2 tablespoons mayo
⅓ cup finely ground pork rinds
1 avocado
Juice of ½ lime

1 Press the Sauté button and press the Adjust button to set heat to Less. Add coconut oil to Instant Pot®. Allow to fully preheat to become nonstick. Remove skin from salmon filet. Finely mince salmon and place in large bowl. Add remaining ingredients except avocado and lime to bowl and form 4 patties.

2 Place burgers into pot and sear each side about 3–4 minutes until center feels firm and reads 145°F on meat thermometer. Press the Cancel button and set aside.

3 Cut open avocado, remove pit, and scoop out flesh. In small bowl, mash avocado with fork and squeeze in juice from lime. Divide mash into four sections and place on top of salmon burgers. Serve warm.

CALORIES: 425	FAT: 27.6 grams
PROTEIN: 35.6 grams	SODIUM: 668 milligrams
FIBER: 2.5 grams	CARBOHYDRATES: 3.8 grams
NET CARBOHYDRATES: 1.3 grams	SUGAR: 0.4 grams

GROUND PORK RINDS

Instead of flours or breadcrumbs, which are high in carbs, you can make a binder using pork rinds. Simply empty the bag into your food processor and pulse until it's a flour or dust consistency. This works great to add crunch to meals or as a binder for meat.

Foil Pack Salmon

Fish can be intimidating because cooking instructions often get confusing. Get ready to prepare perfect salmon easier than ever before. The trick? Tinfoil and your trusty Instant Pot®!

- **Hands-on time:** 2 minutes
- **Cook time:** 7 minutes

Serves 2

2 (3-ounce) salmon filets
1 teaspoon salt
¼ teaspoon pepper
¼ teaspoon garlic powder
¼ teaspoon dried dill
½ lemon
1 cup water

1 Place each filet of salmon skin side down on square of foil. Sprinkle with seasoning and squeeze lemon juice over fish. Slice lemon into four pieces and place two on each filet. Close foil packet by folding over edges.

2 Pour water into Instant Pot® and place steam rack in bottom of pot. Place foil packets on steam rack and click lid closed. Press the Steam button and adjust time for 7 minutes. When timer beeps, quick-release the pressure.

3 Check internal temperature with meat thermometer to ensure thickest part of filet reached at least 145°F. Salmon should easily flake when fully cooked.

CALORIES: 125	**FAT:** 4.6 grams
PROTEIN: 18.5 grams	**SODIUM:** 1,201 milligrams
FIBER: 0.1 grams	**CARBOHYDRATES:** 0.5 grams
NET CARBOHYDRATES: 0.4 grams	**SUGAR:** 0.0 grams

Almond Pesto Salmon

Almonds are a great source of healthy fat. They add the perfect crunch to this dish and give it another layer of flavor. The garlic in the pesto really stands out against the fish and complements the mild flavors of the salmon. This is a great starter recipe for people who are new to seafood or just want something simple and easy.

- **Hands-on time:** 5 minutes
- **Cook time:** 7 minutes

Serves 4

¼ cup sliced almonds
1 tablespoon butter
4 (3-ounce) salmon filets
½ cup pesto
½ teaspoon salt
¼ teaspoon pepper
1 cup water

1 Place almonds and butter into Instant Pot®. Press the Sauté button. Sauté almonds for 3–5 minutes until they begin to soften. Remove and set aside. Press the Cancel button.

2 Brush salmon filets with pesto and add salt and pepper. Pour water into Instant Pot® and place steam rack in bottom. Add salmon to steam rack. Click lid closed. Press the Steam button and adjust time for 7 minutes. Serve warm with almond slices on top.

CALORIES: 182
PROTEIN: 21.2 grams
FIBER: 1.3 grams
NET CARBOHYDRATES: 3.0 grams
FAT: 20.5 grams
SODIUM: 689 milligrams
CARBOHYDRATES: 4.3 grams
SUGAR: 1.3 grams

Cajun Shrimp, Crab, and Sausage Boil

One of the great things about the Instant Pot® is that you can't smell what's cooking until pressure begins to release from the pot. This seafood boil is the perfect meal to use up odds and ends around your kitchen and, it won't leave your home smelling like the sea.

- **Hands-on time: 10 minutes**
- **Cook time: 5 minutes**

Serves 4

½ pound smoked sausage
½ pound shelled deveined large shrimp
2 pounds crab legs
2 cups Seafood Stock (see recipe in Chapter 3)
1 tablespoon Cajun seasoning

Place all ingredients into Instant Pot®. Click lid closed. Press the Steam button and adjust time for 5 minutes. When timer beeps, quick-release the pressure.

CALORIES: 239	FAT: 8.0 grams
PROTEIN: 32.3 grams	SODIUM: 2,139 milligrams
FIBER: 0.0 grams	CARBOHYDRATES: 5.2 grams
NET CARBOHYDRATES: 5.2 grams	SUGAR: 1.1 grams

Steamed Clams

While boiling on the stove may be easy, a clear advantage to using the Instant Pot® is no fishy smell filling your home. Until the pressure starts releasing from the pot, there's generally very little odor. This recipe takes only 10 minutes and won't leave your house smelling like clams for the rest of the day.

- **Hands-on time: 5 minutes**
- **Cook time: 5 minutes**

Serves 4

2 pounds clams
1 cup Seafood Stock (see recipe in Chapter 3)
4 tablespoons butter

Place clams and Seafood Stock into Instant Pot®. Click lid closed. Press the Steam button and adjust time for 5 minutes. When timer beeps, quick-release the pressure. Clams are fully cooked when they naturally open. Serve with butter.

CALORIES: 151	FAT: 11.0 grams
PROTEIN: 8.7 grams	SODIUM: 351 milligrams
FIBER: 0.0 grams	CARBOHYDRATES: 2.1 grams
NET CARBOHYDRATES: 2.1 grams	SUGAR: 0.0 grams

Crispy Blackened Salmon

Salmon is versatile and can complement many flavor profiles. While it's often used with lemon, a Cajun spice rub is just as delicious. This is a perfect Instant Pot® dish because it can be paired with other low-carb sides such as cauliflower rice and only uses one pan. It's great to shake things up and add a bit of kick into your weeknight meal.

- **Hands-on time:** 5 minutes
- **Cook time:** 5 minutes

Serves 2

2 (3-ounce) salmon filets
1 tablespoon avocado oil
1 teaspoon paprika
½ teaspoon salt
¼ teaspoon pepper
¼ teaspoon onion powder
¼ teaspoon dried thyme
⅛ teaspoon cayenne pepper

1 Drizzle avocado oil over salmon. Mix remaining ingredients in small bowl and rub over filets.

2 Press the Sauté button and place salmon into Instant Pot®. Sear 2–5 minutes until seasoning is blackened and easily flakes with fork.

CALORIES: 190
PROTEIN: 18.6 grams
FIBER: 0.6 grams
NET CARBOHYDRATES: 0.5 grams

FAT: 11.4 grams
SODIUM: 620 milligrams
CARBOHYDRATES: 1.1 grams
SUGAR: 0.2 grams

AVOCADO OIL

If you don't have avocado oil, no worries. It can easily be swapped for coconut oil. Avocado has a higher smoke point than other cooking oils (such as olive oil), which allows you to retain the salmon's flavor and health benefits such as supporting healthy blood pressure.

Salmon Stuffed Avocado

It can be hard to figure out what to do with leftover seafood. It's not something you want to leave in the fridge too long but it's hard to get excited about it once it's been reheated. This dish will give life to those leftovers and provide you with a very filling meal.

- **Hands-on time:** 10 Minutes
- **Cook time:** 7 minutes

Serves 2

2 (3-ounce) salmon filets
½ teaspoon salt
¼ teaspoon pepper
1 cup water
⅓ cup mayo
Juice of ½ lemon
2 avocados
½ teaspoon fresh dill, chopped

1 Sprinkle salt and pepper over salmon filets. Pour water into Instant Pot® and place steam rack on bottom.

2 Place salmon skin side down on steam rack. Click lid closed. Press the Steam button and adjust timer for 7 minutes. When timer beeps, quick-release the pressure. Check to make sure salmon is fully cooked, with internal temperature reaching 145°F. Set aside to cool.

3 In large bowl, mix mayo with lemon juice. Cut avocados in half. Remove pits and dice avocados. Add avocados to large bowl and gently fold into mixture.

4 Use fork to flake apart salmon into bite-sized pieces, and gently fold into mixture. Serve garnished with fresh dill.

CALORIES: 602
PROTEIN: 21.5 grams
FIBER: 9.4 grams
NET CARBOHYDRATES: 3.4 grams

FAT: 50.1 grams
SODIUM: 863 milligrams
CARBOHYDRATES: 12.8 grams
SUGAR: 0.8 grams

Fish Taco Bowls

This spicy taco bowl is great for meal prep or when you need to spice things up for dinner. The smoky hints of chili powder in the fish pair well with a creamy slaw. If you're not into spicy, feel free to omit the jalapeños and add your own favorite toppings.

- **Hands-on time:** 15 minutes
- **Cook time:** 5 minutes

Serves 4

4 cups shredded cabbage

¼ cup mayo

2 tablespoons sour cream

1 lime, halved

2 tablespoons chopped pickled jalapeños

3 (4-ounce) tilapia filets

2 teaspoons chili powder

1 teaspoon cumin

1 teaspoon garlic powder

1 teaspoon salt

2 tablespoons coconut oil

1 avocado, diced

4 tablespoons fresh chopped cilantro

1 In large bowl, mix cabbage, mayo, sour cream, juice from half lime, and jalapeños. Cover and place in fridge for at least 30 minutes prior to serving, if possible.

2 Press the Sauté button on Instant Pot®. Pat filets dry and sprinkle evenly with seasonings. Add coconut oil to pot and let melt completely. Add tilapia to pan and sear each side 2–4 minutes or until fully cooked. Fish should flake easily. Press the Cancel button.

3 Chop fish into bite-sized pieces. Separate slaw into four bowls and place fish on top.

4 Cut avocado in half, remove pit, and scoop out flesh. Divide avocado among bowls. Squeeze remaining half of lime juice over dishes and sprinkle with cilantro.

CALORIES: 328	FAT: 23.8 grams
PROTEIN: 19.4 grams	SODIUM: 259 milligrams
FIBER: 4.8 grams	CARBOHYDRATES: 9.0 grams
NET CARBOHYDRATES: 4.2 grams	SUGAR: 2.8 grams

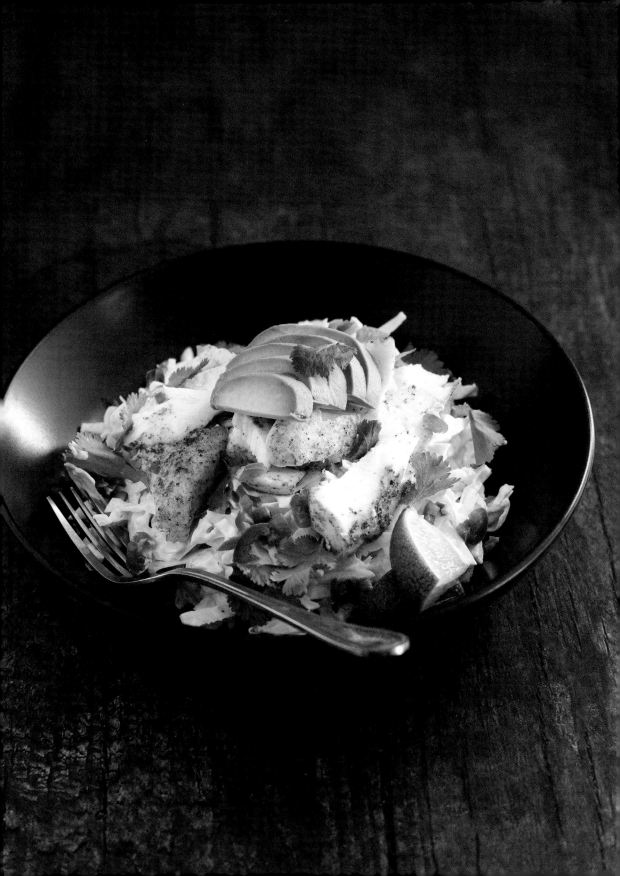

Tomato Cod

Tomato and seafood may seem like an unlikely pair. The mildness of the fish really allows the flavors of the sauce to shine. Cod is a low-fat fish but that doesn't mean you can't enjoy it on a high-fat diet. Just be sure to add plenty of cooking oils and pair it with a fuller-fat side dish to keep things balanced.

- **Hands-on time: 5 minutes**
- **Cook time: 15 minutes**

Serves 4

2 tablespoons butter
¼ cup diced onion
1 clove garlic, minced
1 cup cherry tomatoes
¼ teaspoon salt
⅛ teaspoon pepper
¼ teaspoon dried thyme
¼ cup Chicken Broth (see recipe in Chapter 3)
1 tablespoon capers
4 (4-ounce) cod filets
1 cup water
¼ cup fresh chopped Italian parsley

1 Press the Sauté button and add butter and onions to Instant Pot®. Once onions begin to soften, add garlic and cook additional 30 seconds.

2 Slice tomatoes in half and add to pot with salt, pepper, thyme, and Chicken Broth. Continue cooking sauce for 5–7 minutes or until tomatoes soften. Press the Cancel button.

3 Pour sauce into 7-cup glass bowl. Add capers and fish filets. Cover with foil.

4 Pour water into Instant Pot® and place steam rack on bottom. Place bowl on top. Click lid closed. Press the Manual button and adjust time for 3 minutes. If using a frozen filet, add 2–3 additional minutes.

5 When timer beeps, quick-release the pressure. Sprinkle with fresh parsley and serve.

CALORIES: 157
PROTEIN: 21.0 grams
FIBER: 0.9 grams
NET CARBOHYDRATES: 2.2 grams

FAT: 7.3 grams
SODIUM: 261 milligrams
CARBOHYDRATES: 3.1 grams
SUGAR: 1.5 grams

9

Dessert

Everybody needs their sweets, including people following the keto diet. Thankfully, the Instant Pot® knows how to satisfy your sweet tooth by quickly cooking delicious, low-carb desserts that always hit the spot. You won't have to feel guilty about indulging in the creations from this chapter. From Chocolate Cheesecake to Brownies, you won't believe the decadent, sugar-free recipes that are perfectly acceptable in this way of eating.

Berries and Cream Syrup

This berry syrup is perfect for drizzling on everything from low-carb pancakes, to custard, to cheesecake. Most fruits are typically too high in carbs to be keto-friendly, but berries are generally the exception. This recipe gets you that sweet, tangy, fruity flavor in minutes without going overboard on carbs.

- **Hands-on time:** 2 minutes
- **Cook time:** 4 minutes

Makes 1 cup; serving size 2 tablespoons

1 cup fresh strawberries
1 cup fresh blackberries
½ cup fresh blueberries
2 tablespoons lemon juice
1 tablespoon water
2 tablespoons heavy cream
¼ teaspoon xanthan gum
1 cup water

WHERE DO I USE IT?

This syrup makes the perfect topping drizzled over sugar-free whipped cream or your favorite low-carb yogurt. It can also be swirled into a cheesecake for a burst of tangy flavor without adding many additional carbs.

1. Place all berries, lemon juice, and water into 7-cup glass bowl. Insert steam rack in Instant Pot® and place bowl on top. Add 1 cup water to pot. Click lid closed. Press the Manual button and adjust time for 4 minutes.

2. When timer beeps, quick-release the pressure. Pour berries and juice into food processor or blender. Pulse until smooth. Use fine-mesh strainer to remove seeds and fruit skin from mixture. Whisk in heavy cream and xanthan gum. Keep in sealed container or Mason jar in fridge.

CALORIES: 32	**FAT:** 1.4 grams
PROTEIN: 0.5 grams	**SODIUM:** 1 milligram
FIBER: 1.6 grams	**CARBOHYDRATES:** 4.9 grams
NET CARBOHYDRATES: 3.3 grams	**SUGAR:** 2.9 grams

Slow Cooker Candied Pecans

Candied Pecans are a great addition to everything from rich desserts to fresh salads. Cooking them under pressure in your Instant Pot® with a sugar substitute will give you a great keto-friendly alternative that you can enjoy as an easy snack or store until it's time to top a main dish.

- **Hands-on time: 5 minutes**
- **Cook time: 3 hours**

Makes 2 cups; serving size ¼ cup

2 egg whites
2 cups whole pecans
½ cup powdered erythritol
3 tablespoons melted butter
3 teaspoons cinnamon
1 teaspoon vanilla extract
1 tablespoon water (optional)

TIME MANAGEMENT TIP

This is a great recipe to make while you're cleaning in the kitchen since it requires frequent stirring. When you're in a pinch, these can also make a great gift. Simply add pecans to a small Mason jar and tie a colorful ribbon around the neck of the jar.

1 Whisk egg whites and add remaining ingredients to bowl. Place in Instant Pot® and press the Slow Cook button. You may use a clear slow cooker lid.

2 Place nut mixture into Instant Pot® and stir every 45 minutes for 3 hours until pecans are softened. If they begin sticking to pot, add 1 tablespoon of water when stirring.

CALORIES: 217
PROTEIN: 3.3 grams
FIBER: 2.9 grams
NET CARBOHYDRATES: 1.5 grams
SUGAR ALCOHOLS: 9.0 grams
FAT: 21.0 grams
SODIUM: 14 milligrams
CARBOHYDRATES: 13.4 grams
SUGAR: 1.1 grams

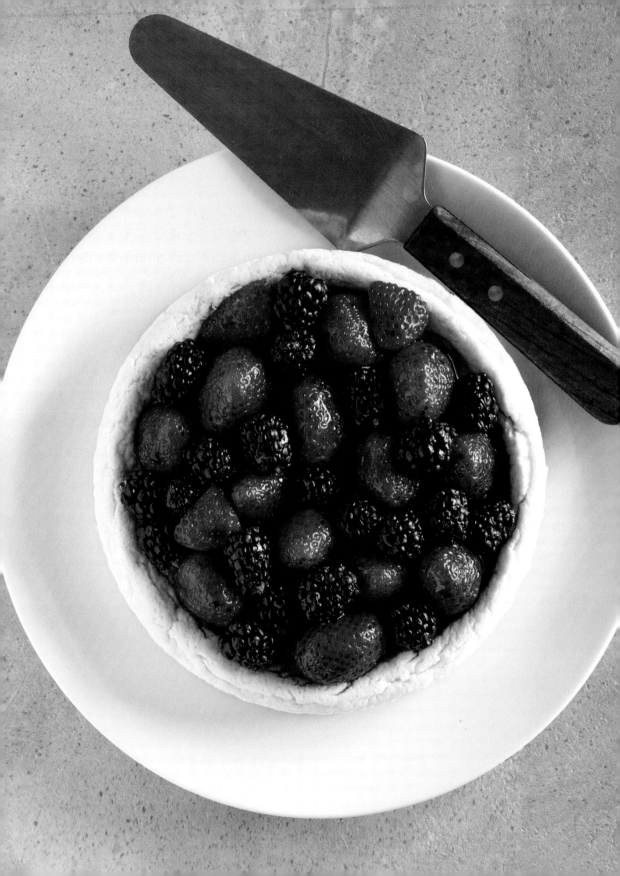

Crustless Berry Cheesecake

This creamy crustless cheesecake is a filling treat to satisfy your after-meal cravings. It's the perfect balance of tartness and richness without feeling overly indulgent. You won't need more than one slice, but you won't have to feel guilty about grabbing another!

- **Hands-on time:** 10 minutes
- **Cook time:** 40 minutes

Serves 12

16 ounces cream cheese, softened

1 cup powdered erythritol

¼ cup sour cream

2 teaspoons vanilla extract

2 eggs

2 cups water

¼ cup blackberries and strawberries for topping

1 In large bowl, beat cream cheese and erythritol until smooth. Add sour cream, vanilla, and eggs and gently fold until combined.

2 Pour batter into 7-inch springform pan. Gently shake or tap pan on counter to remove air bubbles and level batter. Cover top of pan with tinfoil. Pour water into Instant Pot® and place steam rack in pot.

3 Carefully lower pan into pot. Press the Cake button and press the Adjust button to set heat to More. Set time for 40 minutes. When timer beeps, allow a full natural release. Using sling, carefully lift pan from Instant Pot® and allow to cool completely before refrigerating.

4 Place strawberries and blackberries on top of cheesecake and serve.

CALORIES: 153	FAT: 12.7 grams
PROTEIN: 3.4 grams	SODIUM: 152 milligrams
FIBER: 0.1 grams	CARBOHYDRATES: 14.2 grams
NET CARBOHYDRATES: 1.9 grams	SUGAR: 1.7 grams
SUGAR ALCOHOLS: 12.0 grams	

Slow Cooker Mint Hot Chocolate

When the air turns cool, a cup of creamy hot chocolate is the perfect way to end the day. Whether you're entertaining a group or having a family fun night with the kids, this no-fuss drink is the way to go. It has the taste of classic hot chocolate without being loaded with sugar. You can top it with homemade whipped topping, sugar-free chocolate shavings, or cinnamon. Sip slowly and relax knowing this indulgent treat won't derail your goals.

- **Hands-on time: 3 minutes**
- **Cook time: 1 hour**

Serves 4

4 cups unsweetened almond milk

½ cup heavy cream

3 tablespoons unsweetened cocoa powder

½ cup powdered erythritol

¼ cup low-carb chocolate chips

1 teaspoon vanilla extract

½ teaspoon mint extract

Place all ingredients into Instant Pot®, place slow cooker lid on pot, and press the Slow Cook button. Press the Adjust button to set heat to Low and set time for 1 hour. Stir occasionally to help chocolate chips melt and incorporate. Serve warm.

CALORIES: 216	**FAT:** 18.0 grams
PROTEIN: 2.4 grams	**SODIUM:** 172 milligrams
FIBER: 2.5 grams	**CARBOHYDRATES:** 30.4 grams
NET CARBOHYDRATES: 8.2 grams	**SUGAR:** 1.1 grams
SUGAR ALCOHOLS: 19.8 grams	

WHIP IT!

Making low-carb whipped cream is easy. Place ½ cup heavy cream, 1 tablespoon of powdered erythritol, or sweetener of choice, and splash of vanilla in Mason jar and shake until cream forms. Alternatively, place in bowl and beat until fluffy cream forms. If you over whip, you'll end up with sweet butter!

Almond Butter Fat Bomb

"Fat bombs" are a notable part of a keto diet. While they're not necessary for success, they're a helpful way to hit your fat macros to help keep you full. They're also a great way to have a quick and satisfying dessert on this diet. Try these simple nutty and creamy cups if you need a sweet treat!

- **Hands-on time: 3 minutes**
- **Cook time: 3 minutes**

Serves 6

¼ cup coconut oil
¼ cup no-sugar-added almond butter
2 tablespoons cacao powder
¼ cup powdered erythritol

WHAT IS A FAT BOMB?

A fat bomb is a low-carb sweet treat where most of the calories come from fat—usually 70 percent or more. These are used to help fight off hunger, satisfy a sweet tooth, and to help round out your macros for the day.

1 Press the Sauté button and add coconut oil to Instant Pot®. Let coconut oil melt completely and press the Cancel button. Stir in remaining ingredients. Mixture will be liquid.

2 Pour into 6 silicone molds and place into freezer for 30 minutes until set. Store in fridge.

CALORIES: 142 grams
PROTEIN: 2.7 grams
FIBER: 2.0 grams
NET CARBOHYDRATES: 1.4 grams
SUGAR ALCOHOL: 6.0 grams
FAT: 14.1 grams
SODIUM: 33 milligrams
CARBOHYDRATES: 9.4 grams
SUGAR: 0.4 grams

Chocolate Chip Fat Bomb

These Chocolate Chip Fat Bombs will take care of your cookie cravings. They're a sweet, sugar-free treat that will make you believe you're eating cookie dough!

- **Hands-on time:** 2 minutes
- **Cook time:** 2 minutes

Serves 12

½ cup coconut oil
½ cup no-sugar-added peanut butter
2 ounces cream cheese, warmed
¼ cup powdered erythritol
¼ cup low-carb chocolate chips

1 Press the Sauté button and add coconut oil to Instant Pot®. Allow oil to melt and press the Cancel button.

2 Stir in peanut butter, cream cheese, and erythritol. Pour mixture into silicone baking cups or 12-cup muffin tin and sprinkle chocolate chips into each. Place in freezer until firm then keep in fridge.

CALORIES: 181
PROTEIN: 3.0 grams
FIBER: 1.3 grams
NET CARBOHYDRATES: 3.6 grams
SUGAR ALCOHOL: 3.6 grams
FAT: 16.8 grams
SODIUM: 17 milligrams
CARBOHYDRATES: 8.5 grams
SUGAR: 0.8 grams

Chocolate Mousse

This decadent dessert is light but so rich. Serve it in small shot or parfait glasses at your next dinner party.

- **Hands-on time:** 5 minutes
- **Cook time:** 5 minutes

Serves 4

1 cup heavy whipping cream
½ teaspoon gelatin
1 tablespoon erythritol
1 teaspoon vanilla extract
1 cup chocolate pudding

1 In medium bowl, place heavy cream and gelatin. Microwave for 10 seconds and whisk until gelatin is dissolved. Add erythritol and vanilla. Whisk until soft peaks form.

2 Gently fold in chocolate pudding. Serve chilled.

CALORIES: 289
PROTEIN: 2.7 grams
FIBER: 0.0 grams
NET CARBOHYDRATES: 14.8 grams
SUGAR ALCOHOL: 3.0 grams
FAT: 23.2 grams
SODIUM: 109 milligrams
CARBOHYDRATES: 17.8 grams
SUGAR: 11.5 grams

Blackberry Crunch

Sweetness, tartness, and a bit of crunch make this the perfect individual treat. There are many high-carb fruits out there you may love, but berries are generally low-glycemic and can be enjoyed in moderation. Feel free to swap the blackberries for a mix of your other favorite berries and top off with a spoonful of homemade whipped cream.

- **Hands-on time:** 5 minutes
- **Cook time:** 5 minutes

Serves 1

10 blackberries

½ teaspoon vanilla extract

2 tablespoons powdered erythritol

⅛ teaspoon xanthan gum

1 tablespoon butter

¼ cup chopped pecans

3 teaspoons almond flour

½ teaspoon cinnamon

2 teaspoons powdered erythritol

1 cup water

1 Place blackberries, vanilla, erythritol, and xanthan gum in 4-inch ramekin. Stir gently to coat blackberries.

2 In small bowl, mix remaining ingredients. Sprinkle over blackberries and cover with foil. Press the Manual button and set time for 4 minutes. When timer beeps, quick-release the pressure. Serve warm. Feel free to add scoop of whipped cream on top.

CALORIES: 346

PROTEIN: 3.4 grams

FIBER: 8.0 grams

NET CARBOHYDRATES: 5.5 grams

SUGAR ALCOHOL: 24.0 grams

FAT: 30.7 grams

SODIUM: 1 milligram

CARBOHYDRATES: 37.5 grams

SUGAR: 4.8 grams

Peanut Butter Cheesecake Bites

These mini cheesecakes are the perfect size for a family dessert. They're super creamy and so easy to make that the kids can even help. Cheesecake is one of my favorite keto desserts because it can take on so many flavors and forms. You don't have to feel restricted when you're eating something this delicious!

- **Hands-on time:** 10 minutes
- **Cook time:** 15 minutes

Serves 8

16 ounces cream cheese, softened
1 cup powdered erythritol
½ cup peanut flour
¼ cup sour cream
2 teaspoons vanilla extract
2 eggs
2 cups water
¼ cup low-carb chocolate chips
1 tablespoon coconut oil

1 In large bowl, beat cream cheese and erythritol until smooth. Gently fold in peanut flour, sour cream, and vanilla. Fold in eggs slowly until combined.

2 Pour batter into four 4-inch springform pans or silicone cupcake molds. Cover with foil. Pour water into Instant Pot® and place steam rack in pot.

3 Carefully lower pan into pot. Press the Cake button and press the Adjust button to set heat to More. Set time for 15 minutes. When timer beeps, allow a full natural release. Carefully lift cups from Instant Pot® and allow to cool completely before refrigerating.

4 In small bowl, microwave chocolate chips and coconut oil for 30 seconds and whisk until smooth. Drizzle over cheesecakes. Chill in fridge.

CALORIES: 290
PROTEIN: 7.0 grams
FIBER: 1.1 grams
NET CARBOHYDRATES: 6.5 grams
SUGAR ALCOHOL: 18.9 grams

FAT: 22.8 grams
SODIUM: 234 grams
CARBOHYDRATES: 26.5 grams
SUGAR: 2.5 grams

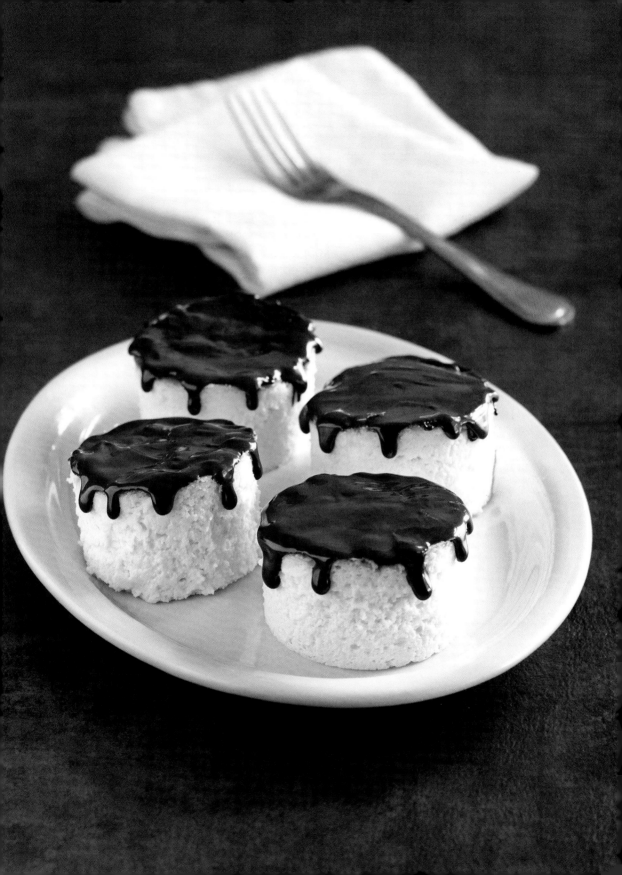

Pecan Clusters

You may be tempted by sugar-free candy at the grocery store, but not all candy is created equal. Many of those use maltitol as a sweetener, which is known to cause tummy trouble. It also has a high glycemic index compared to more ketogenic-friendly sweeteners such as stevia and erythritol. That's why it's so great to make it yourself and know exactly what goes into your treats. If you like pecan pie, you'll enjoy these clusters.

- **Hands-on time:** 5 minutes
- **Cook time:** 5 minutes

Makes 8 clusters; serving size 1 cluster

3 tablespoons butter
¼ cup heavy cream
1 teaspoon vanilla extract
1 cup chopped pecans
¼ cup low-carb chocolate chips

1 Press the Sauté button and add butter to Instant Pot®. Allow butter to melt and begin to turn golden brown. Once it begins to brown, immediately add heavy cream. Press the Cancel button.

2 Add vanilla and chopped pecans to Instant Pot®. Allow to cool for 10 minutes, stirring occasionally. Spoon mixture onto parchment-lined baking sheet to form eight clusters, and scatter chocolate chips over clusters. Place in fridge to cool.

CALORIES: 194
PROTEIN: 1.5 grams
FIBER: 1.8 grams
NET CARBOHYDRATES: 4.0 grams
SUGAR ALCOHOL: 0.9 grams

FAT: 18.2 grams
SODIUM: 3 milligrams
CARBOHYDRATES: 6.7 grams
SUGAR: 0.8 grams

Classic Fudge

Fudge is sweet, smooth, and most important, it doesn't make you feel like you aren't enjoying food when you're on a low-carb diet. With a treat this sweet it's hard to miss sugar and regular chocolate. Just be sure to pick up keto-friendly chocolate chips that are sweetened with a low-glycemic sweetener such as stevia.

- **Hands-on time:** 5 minutes
- **Cook time:** 3 minutes

Makes 10 pieces; serving size 1 piece

1 cup low-carb chocolate chips
8 ounces cream cheese
¼ cup erythritol
¼ teaspoon cinnamon
1 teaspoon vanilla extract
1 cup water

1. Place chocolate chips, cream cheese, erythritol, cinnamon, and vanilla into 7-cup glass bowl. Cover with foil. Place on steam rack inside Instant Pot®. Pour water in bottom of pot.

2. Click lid closed. Press the Manual button and adjust time for 3 minutes. When timer beeps, allow a natural release. When pressure indicator drops, remove bowl carefully and stir ingredients until smooth.

3. Pour mixture into 8" × 8" parchment-lined pan and chill for 2 hours. Slice.

CALORIES: 190
PROTEIN: 1.4 grams
FIBER: 1.6 grams
NET CARBOHYDRATES: 11.0 grams
SUGAR ALCOHOL: 7.6 grams
FAT: 13.9 grams
SODIUM: 82 milligrams
CARBOHYDRATES: 20.2 grams
SUGAR: 0.1 grams

Lemon Poppy Seed Cake

This light cake is perfect for breakfast on a warm, sunny morning. When you work with quality ingredients like almond flour, you don't have to wonder if what you're eating is unhealthy. This cake is perfect for a little treat and the hint of lemon from the zest adds a little tartness to wake the senses.

- **Hands-on time:** 10 minutes
- **Cook time:** 25 minutes

Serves 6

1 cup almond flour
2 eggs
½ cup erythritol
2 teaspoons vanilla extract
1 teaspoon lemon extract
1 tablespoon poppy seeds
4 tablespoons melted butter
¼ cup heavy cream
⅛ cup sour cream
½ teaspoon baking powder
1 cup water
¼ cup powdered erythritol, for garnish

1 In large bowl, mix almond flour, eggs, erythritol, vanilla, lemon, and poppy seeds.

2 Add butter, heavy cream, sour cream, and baking powder.

3 Pour into 7-inch round cake pan. Cover with foil.

4 Pour water into Instant Pot® and place steam rack in bottom. Place baking pan on steam rack and click lid closed. Press the Cake button and press the Adjust button to set heat to Less. Set time for 25 minutes.

5 When timer beeps, allow a 15-minute natural release, then quick-release the remaining pressure. Let cool completely. Sprinkle with powdered erythritol for serving.

CALORIES: 240
PROTEIN: 2.7 grams
FIBER: 2.3 grams
NET CARBOHYDRATES: 3.0 grams
SUGAR ALCOHOL: 22.0 grams

FAT: 20.8 grams
SODIUM: 71 milligrams
CARBOHYDRATES: 27.3 grams
SUGAR: 0.8 grams

Brownies

A dense fudgy brownie with whipped topping is sometimes all you need to wind down for the day. You can relax guilt-free because this dessert is made with sugar-free ingredients and will leave you satisfied without the sugar spike.

- **Hands-on time: 15 minutes**
- **Cook time: 25 minutes**

Serves 6

1 cup low-carb chocolate chips

1 tablespoon coconut oil

1 ounce cream cheese, warmed

¼ cup heavy cream

1 cup almond flour

2 eggs

½ teaspoon baking soda

4 tablespoons melted butter

¾ cup powdered erythritol

1 teaspoon gelatin

½ cup cocoa powder

1 cup water

1 In medium bowl, melt chocolate chips and coconut oil in microwave in 10-second increments until melted and smooth. Set aside.

2 In large bowl, mix cream cheese, heavy cream, almond flour, eggs, baking soda, butter, erythritol, gelatin, and cocoa powder. Fold in melted chocolate.

3 Pour mixture into 7-inch round cake pan and cover with foil. Pour water into Instant Pot® and place steam rack in bottom of pot. Place pan on steam rack and click lid closed. Press the Manual button and adjust time for 25 minutes. When timer beeps, allow a natural release. Serve warm.

CALORIES: 460

PROTEIN: 5.1 grams

FIBER: 7.3 grams

NET CARBOHYDRATES: 20.7 grams

SUGAR ALCOHOL: 22.7 grams

FAT: 35.9 grams

SODIUM: 154 milligrams

CARBOHYDRATES: 50.7 grams

SUGAR: 0.6 grams

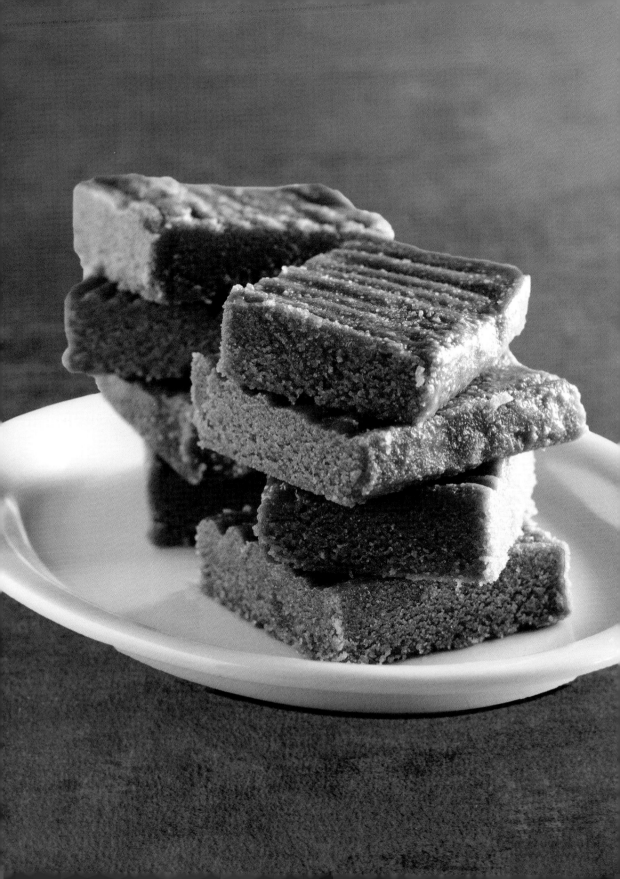

Slow Cooker Peanut Butter Fudge

This fudge is chocolaty with a subtle hint of peanut butter. It's so delicious your friends won't even realize it's sugar-free. Feel free to swap out the peanut butter with your favorite nut butter.

- **Hands-on time: 5 minutes**
- **Cook time: 2 hours**

Makes 12 squares; serving size 1 square

1 cup low-carb chocolate chips
8 ounces cream cheese
¼ cup erythritol
¼ cup no-sugar-added peanut butter
1 teaspoon vanilla extract

1 Place all ingredients into Instant Pot® and cover with slow cooker lid.

2 Allow to cook on Low for 1 hour and stir. Smooth mixture and allow to cook additional 30 minutes.

3 Pour mixture into 8" × 8" parchment-lined pan and chill for 2 hours. Slice.

CALORIES: 159
PROTEIN: 1.9 grams
FIBER: 1.8 grams
NET CARBOHYDRATES: 9.5 grams
SUGAR ALCOHOL: 50.3 grams
FAT: 11.5 grams
SODIUM: 35 milligrams
CARBOHYDRATES: 61.6 grams
SUGAR: 0.7 grams

DESSERTS ON KETO

You can have dessert every day on a keto diet as long as it fits into your macros and calories. Since you do not use sugar or high-carb ingredients, there is no harm in eating a treat every day, if you like. It's a great way to get in extra fat at the end of the day.

Chocolate Pudding

Don't be fooled by the sugar-free pudding cups at the store, as they're often loaded with preservatives and have high-glycemic zero-calorie sweeteners. These may be zero-carb, but they can make you crave sweets. It's better to make your own and know exactly what ingredients you're putting into a dish. This pudding is thick and creamy and will even make the kiddos happy.

- **Hands-on time:** 5 minutes
- **Cook time:** 15 minutes

Serves 4

2 cups unsweetened vanilla almond milk, divided

½ cup heavy cream

2 egg yolks

1 teaspoon vanilla extract

⅛ teaspoon cinnamon

2 tablespoons cocoa powder

¾ teaspoon guar gum

¼ cup low-carb chocolate chips

MAKE SMOOTH PUDDING

If your pudding comes out with some lumps, just run it through a mesh strainer for a smooth consistency.

1 Press the Sauté button and press the Adjust button to set heat to Less. Pour half of almond milk into Instant Pot®. Pour in heavy cream. Bring to gentle boil.

2 In medium bowl, whisk yolks, vanilla, cinnamon, cocoa powder, and guar gum. Slowly whisk into milk mixture and continue quickly whisking until smooth. Press the Cancel button.

3 Add chocolate chips to pot and whisk very quickly until melted. Pour mixture into a large bowl and refrigerate for 2 hours.

CALORIES: 224

PROTEIN: 3.0 grams

FIBER: 2.2 grams

NET CARBOHYDRATES: 8.0 grams

SUGAR ALCOHOL: 1.8 grams

FAT: 18.7 grams

SODIUM: 95 milligrams

CARBOHYDRATES: 12.0 grams

SUGAR: 1.1 grams

Chocolate Cheesecake

Decadent creamy cheesecake is just what you need some days. This cheesecake is rich and perfect for chocolate lovers and special occasions. One of the concerns with cheesecake is cracking, but when you cook in the Instant Pot® you don't have to worry about a water bath for steam. Making cheesecake has never been so easy.

- **Hands-on time: 10 minutes**
- **Cook time: 50 minutes**

Serves 12

2 cups pecans

2 tablespoons butter

16 ounces cream cheese, softened

1 cup powdered erythritol

¼ cup sour cream

2 tablespoons cocoa powder

2 teaspoons vanilla extract

2 cups low-carb chocolate chips

1 tablespoon coconut oil

2 eggs

2 cups water

1 Preheat oven to 400°F. Place pecans and butter into food processor. Pulse until dough-like consistency. Press into bottom of 7-inch springform pan. Bake for 10 minutes then set aside to cool.

2 While crust bakes, mix cream cheese, erythritol, sour cream, cocoa powder, and vanilla together in large bowl using a rubber spatula. Set aside.

3 In medium bowl, combine chocolate chips and coconut oil. Microwave in 20-second increments until chocolate begins to melt and then stir until smooth. Gently fold chocolate mixture into cheesecake mixture.

4 Add eggs and gently fold in, careful not to overmix. Pour mixture over cooled pecan crust. Cover with foil.

5 Pour water into Instant Pot® and place steam rack on bottom. Place cheesecake on steam rack and click lid closed. Press the Manual button and adjust time for 40 minutes. When timer beeps, allow a natural release. Carefully remove and let cool completely. Serve chilled.

CALORIES: 481

PROTEIN: 5.1 grams

FIBER: 4.6 grams

NET CARBOHYDRATES: 19.3 grams

SUGAR ALCOHOL: 16.7 grams

FAT: 38.9 grams

SODIUM: 152 milligrams

CARBOHYDRATES: 40.6 grams

SUGAR: 2.1 grams

Chocolate Mug Cake

This single-serve chocolate treat will get you the dessert you need quicker! Don't worry, this cake is not meant to be shared, so go ahead and indulge...and don't forget to finish it off with a generous dollop of whipped cream, low-carb frosting, or add a couple teaspoons of peanut powder to whipped cream!

- **Hands-on time:** 5 minutes
- **Cook time:** 20 minutes

Serves 1

1 cup water
¼ cup almond flour
2 tablespoons coconut flour
1 egg
2 tablespoons erythritol
½ teaspoon vanilla extract
1 tablespoon butter
2 teaspoons cocoa powder

1 Pour water into Instant Pot®. In medium bowl, mix remaining ingredients. Pour into 4-inch ramekin or oven-safe mug. Cover with foil.

2 Place steam rack into pot and place mug onto steam rack. Click lid closed. Press the Manual button and adjust time for 20 minutes. When timer beeps, allow a natural release. Serve warm.

CALORIES: 384
PROTEIN: 9.1 grams
FIBER: 9.3 grams
NET CARBOHYDRATES: 7.4 grams
SUGAR ALCOHOL: 24.0 grams
FAT: 28.5 grams
SODIUM: 102 milligrams
CARBOHYDRATES: 40.7 grams
SUGAR: 1.5 grams

Vanilla Tea Cake

This cake whips up in just a few minutes and may remind you of pound cake. It's dense yet lightly sweetened so it pairs well with coffee or tea. The trick to this is making sure it's completely cooled before you try to remove it from the pan. Almond flour isn't as sturdy as regular baking flour, but it does firm up the more it cools. Feel free to top your cake with a low-carb frosting, or even just whipped cream!

- **Hands-on time:** 10 minutes
- **Cook time:** 25 minutes

Serves 8

1 cup almond flour
2 eggs
½ cup erythritol
2 teaspoons vanilla extract
4 tablespoons melted butter
¼ cup heavy cream
½ teaspoon baking powder
1 cup water

1 In large bowl, mix all ingredients except water. Pour into 7-inch round cake pan. Cover with foil.

2 Pour water into Instant Pot® and place steam rack in bottom. Place baking pan on steam rack and click lid closed. Press the Cake button and press the Adjust button to set heat to Less. Set time for 25 minutes.

3 When timer beeps, allow a 15-minute natural release, then quick-release the remaining pressure. Let cool completely.

CALORIES: 166
PROTEIN: 1.8 grams
FIBER: 1.5 grams
NET CARBOHYDRATES: 10.0 grams
SUGAR ALCOHOL: 4.0 grams
FAT: 14.6 grams
SODIUM: 51 milligrams
CARBOHYDRATES: 15.5 grams
SUGAR: 0.4 grams

Espresso Cream

All you need are a few spoonfuls of this decadent custard to feel like you're enjoying a treat. Rich creaminess from the egg yolks give it a deep flavor that highlights the espresso. Feel free to add a pinch of cinnamon and a scoop of whipped cream to complete this café-flavored treat.

- **Hands-on time:** 10 minutes
- **Cook time:** 9 minutes

Serves 4

1 cup heavy cream
½ teaspoon espresso powder
½ teaspoon vanilla extract
2 teaspoons unsweetened cocoa powder
¼ cup low-carb chocolate chips
½ cup powdered erythritol
3 egg yolks
1 cup water

1 Press the Sauté button and add heavy cream, espresso powder, vanilla, and cocoa powder. Bring mixture to boil and add chocolate chips. Press the Cancel button. Stir quickly until chocolate chips are completely melted.

2 In medium bowl, whisk erythritol and egg yolks. Fold mixture into Instant Pot® chocolate mix. Ladle into four (4-inch) ramekins.

3 Rinse inner pot and replace. Pour in 1 cup of water and place steam rack on bottom of pot. Cover ramekins with foil and carefully place on top of steam rack. Click lid closed.

4 Press the Manual button and adjust time for 9 minutes. Allow a full natural release. When the pressure indicator drops, carefully remove ramekins and allow to completely cool, then refrigerate. Serve chilled with whipped topping.

CALORIES: 320
PROTEIN: 3.4 grams
FIBER: 1.3 grams
NET CARBOHYDRATES: 8.7 grams
SUGAR ALCOHOL: 19.8 grams
FAT: 28.7 grams
SODIUM: 28 milligrams
CARBOHYDRATES: 29.8 grams
SUGAR: 1.8 grams

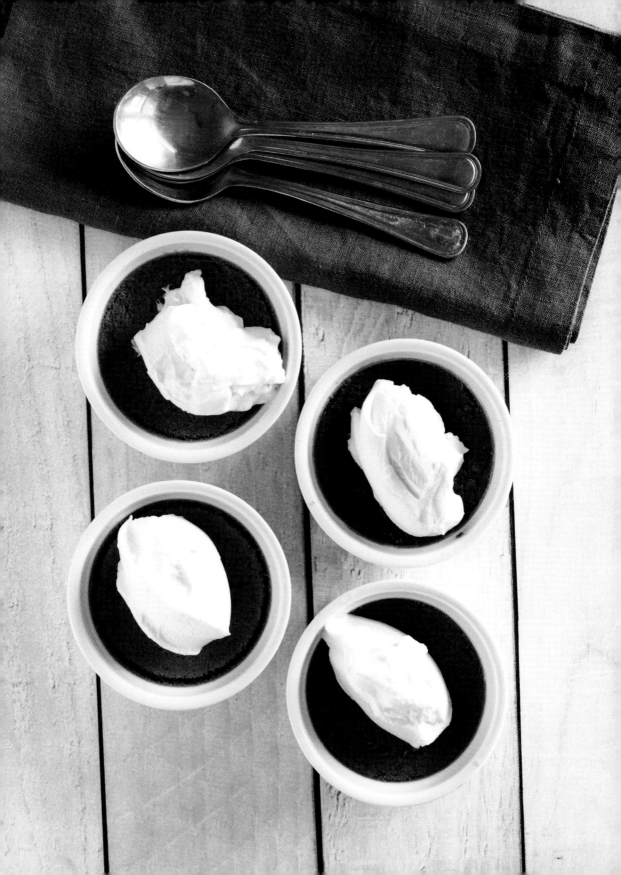

Walnut Crust Pumpkin Cheesecake

Not limited to walnuts, this crust can be made from any of your favorite nuts, such as pecans or almonds. It's got a bit of crunch that adds a wonderful contrast to the creamy cheesecake. You can even make your own pumpkin purée in the Instant Pot®! (See recipe for Fresh Pumpkin Purée in Chapter 5.) If you choose to buy it at the store, be sure not to confuse your pure pumpkin purée with pumpkin pie filling, as that contains added sugar.

- **Hands-on time:** 15 minutes
- **Cook time:** 50 minutes

Serves 6

2 cups walnuts
3 tablespoons melted butter
1 teaspoon cinnamon
16 ounces cream cheese, softened
1 cup powdered erythritol
⅓ cup heavy cream
⅔ cup pumpkin purée
2 teaspoons pumpkin spice
1 teaspoon vanilla extract
2 eggs
1 cup water

1 Preheat oven to 350°F. Add walnuts, butter, and cinnamon to food processor. Pulse until ball forms. Scrape down sides as necessary. Dough should hold together in ball.

2 Press into greased 7-inch springform pan. Bake for 10 minutes or until it begins to brown. Remove and set aside. While crust is baking, make cheesecake filling.

3 In large bowl, stir cream cheese until completely smooth. Using rubber spatula, mix in erythritol, heavy cream, pumpkin purée, pumpkin spice, and vanilla.

4 In small bowl, whisk eggs. Slowly add them into large bowl, folding gently until just combined.

5 Pour mixture into crust and cover with foil. Pour water into Instant Pot® and place steam rack on bottom. Place pan onto steam rack and click lid closed. Press the Cake button and press the Adjust button to set heat to More. Set timer for 40 minutes.

6 When timer beeps, allow a full natural release. When pressure indicator drops, carefully remove pan and place on counter. Remove foil. Let cool for additional hour and then refrigerate. Serve chilled.

CALORIES: 610
PROTEIN: 12.3 grams
FIBER: 3.3 grams
NET CARBOHYDRATES: 7.9 grams
SUGAR ALCOHOL: 24.0 grams

FAT: 54.5 grams
SODIUM: 307 milligrams
CARBOHYDRATES: 35.2 grams
SUGAR: 4.8 grams

US/Metric Conversion Chart

VOLUME CONVERSIONS

US Volume Measure	Metric Equivalent
⅛ teaspoon	0.5 milliliter
¼ teaspoon	1 milliliter
½ teaspoon	2 milliliters
1 teaspoon	5 milliliters
½ tablespoon	7 milliliters
1 tablespoon (3 teaspoons)	15 milliliters
2 tablespoons (1 fluid ounce)	30 milliliters
¼ cup (4 tablespoons)	60 milliliters
⅓ cup	90 milliliters
½ cup (4 fluid ounces)	125 milliliters
⅔ cup	160 milliliters
¾ cup (6 fluid ounces)	180 milliliters
1 cup (16 tablespoons)	250 milliliters
1 pint (2 cups)	500 milliliters
1 quart (4 cups)	1 liter (about)

WEIGHT CONVERSIONS

US Weight Measure	Metric Equivalent
½ ounce	15 grams
1 ounce	30 grams
2 ounces	60 grams
3 ounces	85 grams
¼ pound (4 ounces)	115 grams
½ pound (8 ounces)	225 grams
¾ pound (12 ounces)	340 grams
1 pound (16 ounces)	454 grams

OVEN TEMPERATURE CONVERSIONS

Degrees Fahrenheit	Degrees Celsius
200 degrees F	95 degrees C
250 degrees F	120 degrees C
275 degrees F	135 degrees C
300 degrees F	150 degrees C
325 degrees F	160 degrees C
350 degrees F	180 degrees C
375 degrees F	190 degrees C
400 degrees F	205 degrees C
425 degrees F	220 degrees C
450 degrees F	230 degrees C

BAKING PAN SIZES

American	Metric
8 x 1½ inch round baking pan	20 x 4 cm cake tin
9 x 1½ inch round baking pan	23 x 3.5 cm cake tin
11 x 7 x 1½ inch baking pan	28 x 18 x 4 cm baking tin
13 x 9 x 2 inch baking pan	30 x 20 x 5 cm baking tin
2 quart rectangular baking dish	30 x 20 x 3 cm baking tin
15 x 10 x 2 inch baking pan	30 x 25 x 2 cm baking tin (Swiss roll tin)
9 inch pie plate	22 x 4 or 23 x 4 cm pie plate
7 or 8 inch springform pan	18 or 20 cm springform or loose bottom cake tin
9 x 5 x 3 inch loaf pan	23 x 13 x 7 cm or 2 lb narrow loaf or pâté tin
1½ quart casserole	1.5 liter casserole
2 quart casserole	2 liter casserole

Index